HOW TO CONQUER
BACKACHE

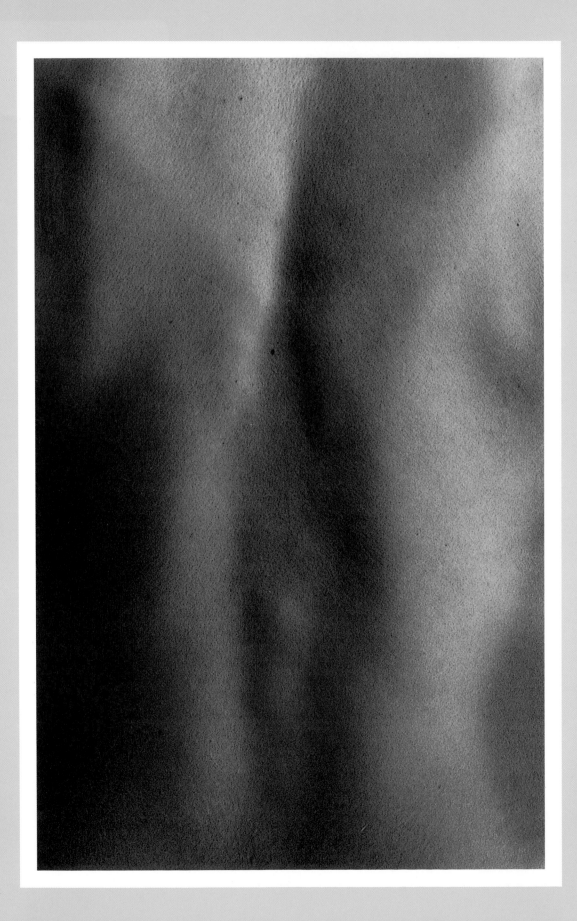

a consultation with **DR VERNON COLEMAN**

HOW TO CONQUER BACKACHE

HAMLYN

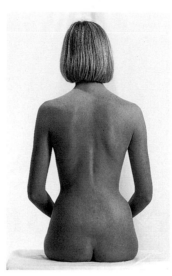

NOTE

THIS BOOK IS NOT INTENDED AS AN ALTERNATIVE TO PERSONAL,
PROFESSIONAL MEDICAL ADVICE. THE READER SHOULD CONSULT A
PHYSICIAN IN ALL MATTERS RELATING TO HEALTH, AND PARTICULARLY IN
RESPECT OF ANY SYMPTOMS WHICH MAY REQUIRE DIAGNOSIS OR MEDICAL
ATTENTION. WHILE THE ADVICE AND INFORMATION ARE BELIEVED TO BE
ACCURATE AND TRUE AT THE TIME OF GOING TO PRESS, NEITHER THE
AUTHOR NOR THE PUBLISHER CAN ACCEPT ANY LEGAL RESPONSIBILITY OR
LIABILITY FOR ANY ERRORS OR OMISSIONS THAT MAY BE MADE

FIRST PUBLISHED IN GREAT BRITAIN 1993
BY HAMLYN, AN IMPRINT OF REED CONSUMER BOOKS LIMITED,
MICHELIN HOUSE, 81 FULHAM ROAD, LONDON SW3 6RB
AND AUCKLAND, MELBOURNE, SINGAPORE AND TORONTO

COPYRIGHT © VERNON COLEMAN 1993
DESIGN AND ILLUSTRATIONS © REED INTERNATIONAL BOOKS LIMITED
1993

ISBN 0 600 57521 7

A CIP RECORD FOR THIS BOOK IS AVAILABLE AT THE BRITISH LIBRARY

PRINTED IN CHINA

CONTENTS

CHAPTER 1 **What Causes Backache**   6

CHAPTER 2 **Slipped Discs**   22

CHAPTER 3 **How To Keep Your Back Healthy**   28

CHAPTER 4 **Exercises For Your Back**   44

CHAPTER 5 **What Doctors Can Do**   70

CHAPTER 6 **Controlling The Pain**   82

CHAPTER 7 **Alternative Solutions**   100

CHAPTER 8 **The Importance Of Relaxation**   110

TWENTY QUESTIONS BACKACHE SUFFERERS OFTEN ASK   118

APPENDIX   124

INDEX   126

CHAPTER ONE

What Causes Backache

Backache is one of the most common of all diseases – and probably the most disabling. Between one-half and three-quarters of adults suffer from it.

In any two week period between one-quarter and one-third of all adults get some back pain. Among 30-, 40- and 50-year olds backache is so common as to be more normal than abnormal.

The pain and the personal agony caused by all this backache is phenomenal but impossible to estimate in any measurable terms, and over the years doctors have made all sorts of attempts to work out just why we suffer so much from backache.

"Backache is one of the most common of all diseases – and probably the most disabling. Between one-half and three-quarters of adults suffer from it."

Back pain first became a real problem when we started standing up and walking around erect, rather than on all fours. If you believe in the creation of man then you will have to put the blame on our maker. But if you believe in evolution you will have to accept that we have not yet evolved far enough to make standing up physiologically sound.

Although the vertebrae – the small bones which make up the spine – fit neatly on top of one another, they were never really designed for an upright posture. The spine is strong enough to withstand pressures of several hundred pounds and is so flexible that it can be bent to form two-thirds of a circle, but the intricate system of muscles, tendons and ligaments which keep the whole thing together can easily be damaged or disrupted in all sorts of ways. The spine acts as a scaffolding for the whole of the body with the skull, ribs, pelvis and limbs attached to it. Through its middle runs the extremely delicate spinal cord – so delicate that even a relatively slight physical abnormality can cause awful pains. While a serious structural problem can cause paralysis and disablement.

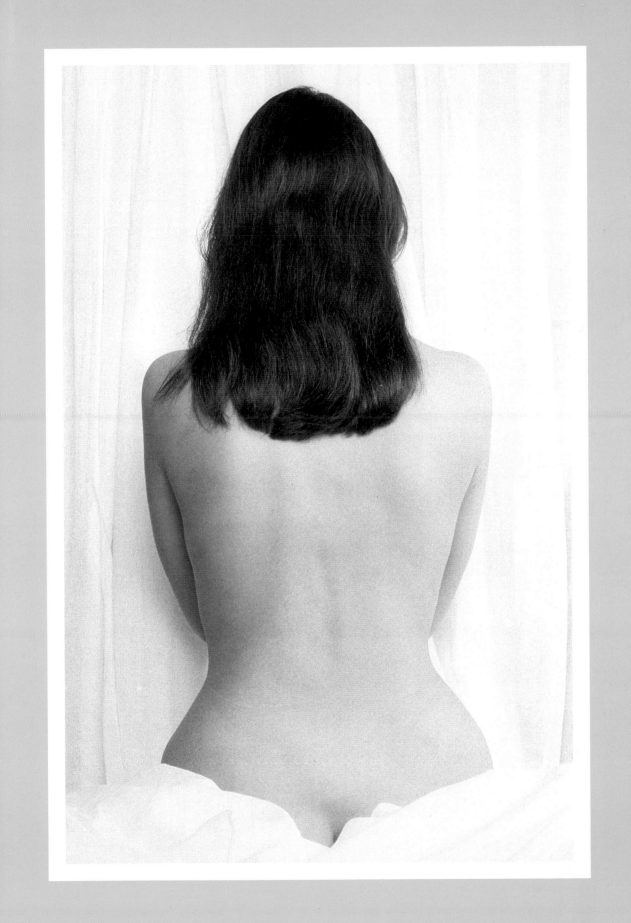

One of the most common causes of back pain is a slipped or prolapsed disc and it really isn't difficult to understand why this causes so much trouble.

It is the bones of the spine which give the back its strength. But if the spine only consisted of bone then you wouldn't be able to bend to tie up your shoe laces or to pick things up off the floor. So between the bones there are 23 intervertebral discs which act as bendy shock absorbers.

The outer part of each disc is tough and rather rubbery but inside that there is a soft, squashy area called the nucleus pulposus (85 per cent of each disc is made up of water). It is this central soft part of the disc that gives us the ability to touch our toes.

When you are lying in bed at night the disc expands and sucks in water and food. But when you are walking or carrying something heavy the bones compress the discs and squeeze out much of the fluid. During the average sort of day most of us lose about a centimetre in height because our discs are compressed. You gain that lost height again every night.

In addition to giving the spine strength the vertebrae also provide essential protection for the spinal cord – the body's biggest nerve. The spinal cord carries impulses from the brain to the arms, legs and body, and then carries messages back from those areas to keep the brain informed.

Hundreds of individual nerves connect the spinal cord to the various parts of the human body.

If the spinal cord is damaged then paralysis will result – the precise nature of the paralysis depending on the place where the spinal cord is damaged.

YOUR SPINE

Your spine is made up of 26 separate bones or vertebrae though two of these consist of several small vertebral bones fixed together. All these bones fit one on top of the other like a pile of children's building bricks. The bones at the top of the spine – where the skull fits on top – are smallest, while the bones at the bottom – where they fit into the bones of the pelvis – are largest. Right at the bottom of spine is the sacrum (which is made up of the sacral vertebrae) and then the coccyx (which is also made up of bones which are normally joined together).

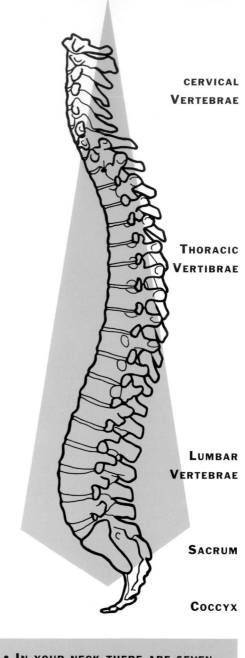

CERVICAL
VERTEBRAE

THORACIC
VERTIBRAE

LUMBAR
VERTEBRAE

SACRUM

COCCYX

- **IN YOUR NECK THERE ARE SEVEN CERVICAL VERTEBRAE**

- **SUPPORTING YOUR CHEST THERE ARE 12 THORACIC VERTEBRAE**

- **NEXT ARE FIVE LUMBAR VERTEBRAE**

- **BELOW THEM IS THE SACRUM (WHICH CONSISTS OF FIVE SACRAL VERTEBRAE)**

- **FINALLY, COMES THE COCCYX OR 'VESTIGIAL TAIL' WHICH CONSISTS OF FOUR TINY VERTEBRAE**

Although I have said that these bones in your back are balanced one on top of the other like a pile of building bricks there is one very important difference: your spine is not straight.

Indeed, it has no less than *four* separate curves which are there to make your spine more capable of coping with stresses and strains:

- **AT THE TOP OF THE SPINE THE CERVICAL VERTEBRAE CURVE FORWARDS**

- *BELOW THEM THE THORACIC VERTEBRAE CURVE BACKWARDS*

- *THE LUMBAR VERTEBRAE CURVE FORWARDS AGAIN*

- *FINALLY THE SACRAL AND COCCYGEAL REGIONS CURVE BACKWARDS*

THE VERTEBRAE – THE BUILDING BLOCKS IN YOUR BACK

Because they vary in size your vertebrae are all different, but there are some important similarities between the majority of them. At the front of each one there is a solid block of bone called the 'body' of the vertebra. The more complicated part of the vertebral bone is at the back and is called the 'neural arch'. This has a hole in the middle of it through which the spinal cord runs, and has a number of bits sticking out of it:

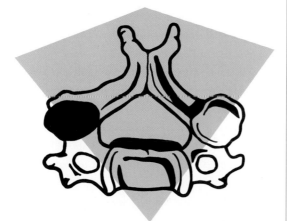

- **TWO 'TRANSVERSE PROCESSES' STICK OUT FROM THE SIDES OF EACH NEURAL ARCH**

- *A 'SUPERIOR ARTICULAR PROCESS' POINTS UPWARDS*

- *AN 'INFERIOR ARTICULAR PROCESS' POINTS DOWNWARDS*

- *AND FROM THE BACK OF EACH NEURAL ARCH THE 'SPINOUS PROCESS' STICKS OUT (THESE ARE THE BONY BITS YOU CAN FEEL IF YOU RUN YOUR FINGERS UP AND DOWN YOUR SPINE).*

HOW ALL THE BONES HOLD TOGETHER

Each of the vertebrae in your spine connects to the one above it and below it. Consider the fourth thoracic vertebra, for example. Above, the 'superior articular process' fits onto the 'inferior articular process' of the third thoracic vertebra, and below, the 'inferior articular process' fits onto the 'superior articular process' of the fifth thoracic vertebra.

It is this series of joints which gives your spine its bony strength. These are not, however, the only joints holding your spine together. There are, altogether, nearly 150 joints in your spine. Right at the top your first cervical vertebra is joined onto the bottom of your skull. And at the bottom of your spine the sacral bones are joined onto your hip bones.

The 12 ribs which give your chest strength and which protect your lungs and heart are attached to your thoracic vertebrae. Without them you would collapse on the floor if you were bumped just as easily as a pile of building bricks falls over if nudged.

IN BETWEEN THE BONES – THE DISCS WHICH ENABLE YOU TO MOVE AND BEND

If your spine consisted only of bone it would be very stiff and immobile. But unless there is something wrong with it your spine is remarkably bendy. There are two things which make this possible.

First, there is the shape of the bones. Your first cervical vertebra (which is also called the 'atlas' bone) allows your head to nod backwards and forwards, and to tilt sideways. Your second cervical vertebra (also known as the 'axis' bone) allows your head to turn to the left and to the right. The other bones of the spine also allow a certain amount of backward, forward and sideways movement.

More important even than the shape of your bones are the 'intervertebral discs' – the 23 narrow spongy shock absorbers which fit between the 24 separate bones of your spine. Without the discs these bones would grate and crunch every time you moved. Each disc has a strong fibrous outer casing – called the annulus fibrosus – and a soft, squashy, jelly-like interior – called the nucleus pulposus – which is reinforced with strands of fibre.

Intervertebral discs have very little in the way of nerve supply and contain no blood. They are made up largely of water. As you get older the amount of fluid in your discs will diminish slightly – and as a result you will get shorter.

LIGAMENTS WHICH GIVE YOUR SPINE ADDED STRENGTH

Wherever two bones come together in your body to produce a joint, the ends of the bones will be held together by strong, slightly elastic fibrous bands called ligaments. The fibres of each of these ligaments lie in the direction of the force that occurs in and around each joint, and by holding the bones firmly together the ligaments make sure that the movement of the joint is properly controlled. The joints of the spine – like all the other joints in your body – are strengthened and protected by ligaments.

THE MUSCLES OF YOUR BACK

Your body contains two types of muscle: involuntary and voluntary.

Involuntary muscles are the sort that do their job quietly and without any prompting. They will carry on for as long as you are alive without you ever being aware of them – unless something goes wrong. Your

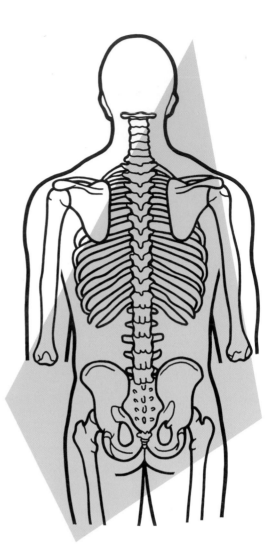

heart is made of involuntary muscle, and your intestines and your blood vessels are surrounded by involuntary muscles.

Voluntary muscles, on the other hand, are largely under your control. The muscles in your fingers and feet and arms and legs are made of voluntary muscles and, by and large, unless you tell them to do something they will stay quiet and immobile. You do not have to tell each muscle what to do, of course. All you have to do is send a message down saying 'cross your knees' or 'start walking', and your muscles will do the rest all by themselves for they are equipped with an amazingly sophisticated system of nerves and reflexes. Sometimes your voluntary muscles can respond to stimuli well before your brain has had time to react. So, for example, if you tread on a nail your muscles will move your foot away from the source of the pain automatically and without any need for your brain to intervene.

Whatever type they are, the muscles around your body all consist of long thin fibres which are supplied with their own nerves and blood vessels, and are wrapped up in neat bundles by connective tissue.

Because they can be controlled voluntary muscles can be trained and developed, and with the right sort of exercise you can make your voluntary muscles stronger and bigger. You can also teach them how to respond more quickly and more precisely to nerve messages, and you can build them up so that they obtain oxygen and food supplies more speedily and get rid of waste products more quickly, too. The right sort of training can build up your voluntary muscles in a quite dramatic fashion, though it is, of course, also true that if you do not exercise your muscles properly they will waste away and become small and weak.

The bones of your spine are controlled by two main sets of muscles: those in your back and in your abdomen. (Although the muscles in your neck also have a vital role to play in helping your spine remain well supported and in good health.)

The muscles in your back are divided into two groups – with your spine in the middle. No muscles cross over the vertebral column, and the muscles are fixed to the transverse processes and spinal processes of the vertebrae. You have two matching sets of back muscles: with the superficial muscles being large and sheet-like, and the underlying, deeper muscles being long, strap-like and running almost vertically alongside your spine. The innermost layers of muscles are quite short and thick, and their job is simply to connect each vertebra with its neighbours.

If your back is to remain healthy and erect it is essential that these muscles are all kept strong and in good condition by some form of regular exercise. Unfortunately, most of us spend much of our time sitting down in badly-designed chairs and allowing our muscles to weaken and atrophy. It is hardly surprising that backache is endemic.

The various muscles in your back have the vital role of keeping your spine upright, but they share this responsibility with the muscles in your abdomen which help to provide a counterbalancing force. The muscles in your abdomen also help you to bend and to twist.

YOUR SPINAL CORD AND SPINAL CANAL

The spinal canal isn't really a canal. In reality it is nothing more than a series of holes in the 24 neural arches of the vertebrae. Despite this misnomer the spinal canal is vitally important, for it provides a safe passage for the spinal cord – a massive group of nerves which enables your brain to send and receive messages to and from the rest of your body.

Your spinal cord does not just lie loosely inside your spinal canal but is wrapped in a triple-membrane-layered tube and, like the brain, protected by a layer of cerebro-spinal fluid.

All this protection means that your spinal cord is not especially vulnerable unless your vertebrae are damaged, broken or dislocated. The combination of bone, ligaments, muscle, membranes and fluid look after your spinal cord well, and there is enough room within the spinal canal for the cord to move around when you bend your back.

The protection is essential because from in between every pair of vertebrae nerves leave the spinal cord and create a local network of smaller nerves, which then supply all the local tissues, providing instructions for muscles that your brain wants moving, and sending a constant series of messages to your brain when your various nerve endings pick up new or valuable information.

THE CAUSES OF BACKACHE

Your back is strong enough to withstand pressures of several hundred pounds, and it is so flexible that it can be bent to form two-thirds of a circle. Your spine acts as a scaffolding for the whole of your body to which the skull, ribs, pelvis and limbs are all attached. But the intricate system of bones, muscles, tendons and ligaments which keep the whole thing together can easily be damaged – and there are many possible causes of back pain from *outside* the spine.

Overleaf are some of the most common causes of back trouble. Do note that some are not a result of bone, muscle or joint injury – and some back pain symptoms denote serious underlying problems.

NEVER try to diagnose or treat your own back pain
ALWAYS see a doctor first for advice and help.

NECK:

WHIPLASH SYNDROME. IF YOUR HEAD IS BENT BACKWARDS OR FORWARDS VIOLENTLY YOUR NECK LIGAMENTS CAN BE STRAINED. (LIGAMENTS ARE TOUGH, INELASTIC FIBRES WHICH HOLD BONES TOGETHER.) THE SYMPTOMS ARE PAIN AND STIFFNESS WHICH USUALLY BEGIN SEVERAL HOURS AFTER THE OCCURRENCE OF THE INJURY.

A STIFF NECK THAT IS ACCOMPANIED BY A SEVERE HEADACHE, VOMITING, CONFUSION, DROWSINESS AND A HATRED OF BRIGHT LIGHTS MAY MEAN MENINGITIS (AN INFLAMMATION OF THE MEMBRANE COVERING THE BRAIN AND SPINAL CORD).

A SLIPPED OR PROLAPSED DISC IN THE CERVICAL SPINE COULD RESULT IN A SEVERE PAIN IN YOUR SHOULDER, ARM OR HAND. SMALL MOVEMENTS MAY MAKE THE PAIN WORSE.

BACK AND SHOULDER PAIN WHICH IS MADE WORSE BY BREATHING AND ACCOMPANIED BY A COUGH AND HIGH TEMPERATURE MAY BE CAUSED BY A CHEST INFECTION SUCH AS PNEUMONIA OR PLEURISY.

PAIN AND STIFFNESS IN THE BACK ACCOMPANIED BY NUMBNESS OR TINGLING IN THE FINGERS MAY SUGGEST OSTEOARTHRITIS IN THE BONES OF THE SPINE.

MID BACK:

BACK PAIN THAT BECOMES WORSE AFTER SITTING IN ONE POSITION FOR A LONG TIME MAY BE CAUSED BY POOR POSTURE OR A BADLY-DESIGNED CHAIR.

STRESS, ANXIETY AND EMOTIONAL

WORRIES CAN LEAD TO MUSCLE TENSION WHICH RESULTS IN ACHES AND PAINS IN THE BACK. THIS IS ONE OF THE MOST COMMON CAUSES OF BACK PAIN – PROBABLY AFFECTING AS MANY AS EIGHT OUT OF TEN SUFFERERS.

A SHARP PAIN THAT IS WORSE WHEN YOU BREATHE IN OR MOVE AND WHICH FOLLOWS AN INJURY MAY BE A RESULT OF A BROKEN RIB – OR EVEN A DAMAGED BONE IN THE SPINE.

IF YOUR PAIN STARTED AFTER A TRIVIAL MOVEMENT – SUCH AS TYING UP YOUR SHOE LACES OR TURNING OVER IN BED – IT MAY BE A RESULT OF A SLIPPED DISC OR A JOINT PROBLEM IN YOUR SPINE.

SEVERE, CONSTANT PAIN THAT RADIATES ROUND INTO YOUR CHEST MAY BE A RESULT OF A FRACTURE CAUSED BY OSTEOPOROSIS OR THIN BONES.

PAIN HERE THAT IS ACCOMPANIED BY DISCOMFORT WHEN PASSING URINE, AND/OR BLOOD IN YOUR URINE MAY BE A RESULT OF A KIDNEY INFECTION.

IF YOU GET SEVERE PAIN HERE THAT COMES AND GOES – AND RADIATES DOWN INTO YOUR GROIN – YOU MAY HAVE A KIDNEY STONE.

PAIN IN THE MIDDLE OF THE BACK THAT IS MADE WORSE BY EATING AND ACCOMPANIED BY INDIGESTION MAY SUGGEST A STOMACH ULCER.

A PAIN THAT FOLLOWS STRENUOUS EXERCISE MAY SUGGEST A TORN OR STRAINED MUSCLE.

GENERAL BACKACHE THAT IS MADE WORSE BY MOVEMENT OR COLD WEATHER MAY SUGGEST ARTHRITIS IN THE SPINE.

LOW BACK:

DID YOUR LOW BACK PAIN START FAIRLY QUICKLY AFTER TWISTING, BENDING OR LIFTING OR DID IT OCCUR AFTER SOME APPARENTLY TRIVIAL MOVEMENT? IF SO, THEN IT MAY BE CAUSED BY A SLIPPED OR PROLAPSED DISC.

IF, IN ADDITION TO BACK PAIN, YOU ALSO HAVE PAIN GOING DOWN ONE OR BOTH LEGS, OR NUMBNESS OR TINGLING IN ONE OR BOTH LEGS, THEN YOU MAY BE SUFFERING FROM SCIATICA – IN WHICH THE SCIATIC NERVE CAN BE DAMAGED BY A SLIPPED OR PROLAPSED DISC.

IF YOU ARE UNDER 30 AND YOU FIND THAT YOUR PAIN AND STIFFNESS ARE RELIEVED BY EXERCISE YOU MAY HAVE A CONDITION KNOWN AS ANKYLOSING SPONDYLITIS IN WHICH THE DISCS AND LIGAMENTS OF THE SPINE BECOME STIFF AND BONELIKE.

LOW BACK PAINS THAT ARE ACCOMPANIED BY GYNAECOLOGICAL SYMPTOMS (DISCHARGE, BLEEDING ETC.) MAY SUGGEST A GYNAECOLOGICAL CAUSE – SUCH AS PERIOD PAIN.

BOTTOM OF SPINE:

PAIN IN ONE BUTTOCK – POSSIBLY ACCOMPANIED BY PAIN IN THE BACK OF THE THIGH – MAY BE CAUSED BY A SACROILIAC JOINT STRAIN.

HIP:

PAIN THAT IS MAINLY IN THE HIP OR GROIN, GOES DOWN THE FRONT OF YOUR LEG AND GETS WORSE WHEN YOU WALK MAY BE CAUSED BY AN OSTEOARTHRITIC HIP.

DISEASES THAT CAN AFFECT YOUR SPINE

Not all types of backache are caused by injury, degeneration or old age. There are numerous individual disorders which can affect your spine.

OSTEOARTHRITIS

Probably the most common cause of back pain, osteoarthritis usually first affects older people in their fifties or sixties. It seems to affect women slightly more often than men, and in addition to the joints of the spine usually also affects the knees, hips, hands and feet. To start with there is usually only one joint that suffers but as time goes by osteoarthritis can spread to many parts of the body.

The main symptoms are stiffness and aching which develop as the cartilage between the bones gradually gets thinner and thinner. Eventually the bones end up rubbing on one another.

Osteoarthritis can be caused by excess wear and tear (in which case it is practically indistinguishable from the problems often caused by old age), but it can be inherited and may affect younger adults.

RHEUMATOID ARTHRITIS

There is little doubt that rheumatoid arthritis is one of the most common of all crippling, long-term diseases. Although it usually affects the smaller joints – particularly those of the hands, wrists and feet – it can also be present in the joints of the spine. However, the spine is usually the last part of the body to be attacked and by then other joints will probably be affected. The neck is usually the first part of the spine to be involved.

The initial symptoms are usually pain, tenderness, swelling and stiffness of the joints. These symptoms, which can arrive quite suddenly or which may develop slowly over a long period of time, are nearly always worse first thing in the morning.

Many joints can get rheumatoid arthritis and sufferers who have the disease badly may complain that their whole bodies hurt. The pain and aching is often also accompanied by a general feeling of tiredness, listlessness and of being run down. The symptoms of rheumatoid arthritis are unusual in that they may sometimes disappear for months or years almost completely without any warning – though, sadly, they usually do come back again in the end.

The basic cause of rheumatoid arthritis is still a mystery. One theory is that the disease is caused by a virus, another that it is caused by a flaw in the body's own defence mechanism against infection. It is also generally believed that stress in its many different forms makes rheumatoid arthritis worse.

OSTEOPOROSIS

Osteoporosis affects all the bones – not just the ones of the back – but the first symptoms of osteoporosis often involve the back simply because the vertebrae are under such an enormous amount of pressure.

No one really knows exactly why osteoporosis develops (although it is known that people who exercise regularly are far less likely to suffer from it, and it is also known that in women there is a link to sex hormones since women who have gone through the menopause are far more likely to suffer from it), but calcium and other minerals which are essential for healthy bones leak out, leaving the bones weak and more than usually liable to fracture.

Most people with osteoporosis have smaller vertebrae (with the result that they shrink and become shorter), and it is fairly common for several vertebrae to fracture with the result that the spine eventually becomes noticeably rounded.

Osteoporosis is normally associated with increasing age, but it can be caused by spending long periods in bed – and is, therefore, common among patients suffering from other disorders. It is because of the danger of osteoporosis developing that most doctors like their patients to get up and out of bed as early as possible.

The loss of bone material that occurs in osteoporosis is not painful in itself but the fractures of the bones that result from osteoporosis often are – particularly if nerves are trapped.

OSTEOMALACIA

Osteomalacia is similar to osteoporosis but in this case the softening and weakening of the bones is caused by vitamin D deficiency which affects the body's ability to absorb calcium and phosphorus. When it affects children osteomalacia is called rickets.

ANKYLOSING SPONDYLITIS

Ankylosing spondylitis is the third most common arthritic disease (after osteoarthritis and rheumatoid arthritis). It runs in families and almost (but not completely) exclusively affects young white males between the ages of 15 and 25 years old.

The condition is caused when excessive calcium deposits are laid down, with the results that bones become fused together and ligaments become inflamed and eventually calcify. The spine – particularly the lower back – is the part of the body most commonly affected but other large joints can be hit too, and there is nearly always some general illness.

After some time, if enough joints are affected, the whole of the spine can become rigid or ankylosed, with the result that the sufferer cannot bend. The ligaments which join the vertebrae onto the ribs may also harden with the result that the rib cage becomes flatter and the patient finds it difficult to breathe. Most sufferers also have inflammation of their eyes.

The symptoms of ankylosing spondylitis are pain and stiffness in the back and other affected joints, and although these symptoms are usually worse in the mornings or after any rest or lack of movement they are often relieved by gentle exercise.

ARACHNOIDITIS

The arachnoid is one of the three membranes surrounding the spinal cord and the nerve roots, and arachnoiditis is an inflammation of this membrane. Normally this membrane is thin and pliable but in arachnoiditis the membrane becomes thicker and thicker, gradually squeezing and compressing the nerves so that they can no longer move freely. The inevitable result is pain, though the pain depends upon which nerves have been affected.

There are several possible ways in which arachnoiditis can develop. Sometimes it develops as a result of spinal surgery, and sometimes as a result of an infection of the membranes surrounding the brain and spinal cord (meningitis).

In the past it was not unknown for arachnoiditis to develop after X-rays of the spine in which contrast dyes were used. These are now known to cause inflammation and are no longer used.

PAGET'S DISEASE

Also known as osteitis deformans, Paget's Disease can start in any bone in the body. It is rare before the age of 60. The disease involves the thickening of the bones but instead of becoming tougher and stronger the bones, paradoxically, become softer and tend to deform easily. If Paget's Disease affects the bone of the spine nerves are often compressed – producing pain.

OTHER CAUSES OF BACK PAIN

A problem in your back can cause pain elsewhere in your body. If a nerve in the lower part of your spine is compressed then you may experience a pain in your buttocks, thighs or legs.

Similarly, just because you have a pain in your back there isn't *necessarily* anything wrong with the bones, muscles, joints or ligaments of your back!

You should never assume that your problem must be in your spine just because you have a pain in your back. If you visit your doctor complaining of backache he will probably do all sorts of tests to try and find out what is causing your problem before he concludes that you have a physical back problem.

Here are some of the disorders which can give rise to aches and pains in and around your back:

VIRUS INFECTION

Viruses such as those which cause influenza can cause a wide range of symptoms. Apart from problems such as sore throat, stuffy nose and cough, you may suffer from nausea or a loss of appetite. And you may also notice aches and pains in or around your spine. Pains in the lower back are particularly common with a number of virus infections.

STRESS

Pressure, tension and anxiety can all cause tense muscles. And muscles which are tense can easily go into spasm and become painful. Once a back pain does develop the stress caused by the pain can make things worse – producing extra anxiety which then causes more muscle tension and makes the pain even worse. In four out of every five cases of back pain doctors never find out what has caused the pain – there are no

15

physical abnormalities, not even on X-ray examination. Even family doctors and back pain specialists admit that something like eight out of every ten cases of back pain aren't caused by any genuine physical abnormality but by stress and worry, and by pressure and tension on muscles and joints.

IRRITABLE BOWEL SYNDROME

The irritable bowel syndrome is, without a doubt, one of the most common and most troublesome of all diseases – and it is a common cause of backache.

Amazingly, as many as one in three people suffer from irritable bowel syndrome. It affects men as well as women, and the young as well as the old (though it primarily affects young women in their twenties, thirties and forties).

For the vast majority of sufferers there are three basic symptoms:

- **PAIN – USUALLY COLICKY AND SPASMODIC**
- **DIARRHOEA OR CONSTIPATION**
- **WIND**

But those are by no means the only symptoms. Sufferers also commonly complain of:

- **CONSTANTLY FEELING FULL**
- **NAUSEA, HEARTBURN OR INDIGESTION**
- **URINARY FREQUENCY**
- **TIREDNESS**
- **ANXIETY AND DEPRESSION**
- **BACKACHE**

You should visit your doctor for a precise diagnosis if you suffer from the above and think you could have irritable bowel syndrome.

There are two very common causes. The first is stress. Muscles of all kinds respond dramatically to tension. Headaches, for example, are frequently caused when the muscles around the head are tightened by worry and anxiety. The bowel muscles are as vulnerable as any other.

The second cause is diet. Most of us eat a modern-day diet which is bland and contains far too little natural roughage.

Although we know a good deal about the causes of irritable bowel syndrome we still don't know how to *cure* it; but it can be controlled.

GYNAECOLOGICAL PROBLEMS

Of the many gynaecological problems which can cause back pain the following are among the most common:

DYSMENORRHOEA (PAINFUL PERIODS)

Pain produced during menstruation is usually caused by the uterine contractions which have been triggered by hormonal changes. This sort of pain is usually colicky, starting a few hours before a period arrives, lasting for about a day and often being accompanied by nausea, sweating, fainting and constipation. The pain is usually situated in the lower part of the abdomen, the thighs and the buttocks, but it can also affect the lower part of the back. Simple painkillers such as aspirin and paracetamol may help, and heat applied locally is often extremely effective, but many women obtain most relief by using hormone pills which must, of course, be prescribed by a doctor.

FIBROIDS

The normal, healthy uterus is made up of a large number of powerful muscle fibres. Although no one really knows why they do it these fibres can occasionally grow too much – forming huge muscle tumours commonly known as fibroids.

Benign, and more of a nuisance than a real threat, fibroids are usually fairly small (about the size of a plum) but can grow quite large (up to the size of a grapefruit) and if they are big enough or there are enough of them they can enlarge a woman's abdomen to make her look pregnant.

About one in five women end up growing fibroids and these can produce a wide range of different types of pain – including backache. A surgical operation to remove the fibroids is often the only way to deal permanently with the problem.

RETROVERTED UTERUS

Under normal circumstances the uterus is bent slightly forward, resting on the bladder and lying at an angle of 90° to the vagina. Sometimes, however, the uterus is bent backwards – known as retroversion. It is not dangerous but some doctors believe that it causes backache and may make it difficult for a woman to conceive.

WAYS TO CONQUER
IRRITABLE BOWEL SYNDROME

1. VISIT YOUR DOCTOR.

2. PEPPERMINT OIL CAPSULES ARE EXTREMELY EFFECTIVE AT CONTROLLING THE WIND THAT IS A COMMON SYMPTOM IN SUFFERERS. YOU CAN BUY THESE AT A PHARMACY OR YOU CAN OBTAIN THEM WITH A DOCTOR'S PRESCRIPTION.

3. TRY TO CONTROL THE AMOUNT OF UNNECESSARY STRESS AND PRESSURE IN YOUR LIFE. MAKE A LIST OF THE DIFFERENT PRIORITIES IN YOUR LIFE AND DECIDE HOW YOU ARE GOING TO ALLOCATE YOUR TIME MORE EFFICIENTLY.

4. GRADUALLY INCREASE THE AMOUNT OF FIBRE YOU EAT. EAT WHOLEMEAL BREAD OR HIGH-BRAN CEREALS, WHOLEWHEAT PASTA, BROWN RICE AND FRESH VEGETABLES AND FRUIT. (DO THIS GRADUALLY – IF YOU INCREASE THE AMOUNT OF FIBRE TOO QUICKLY YOU MAY SUFFER FROM *MORE* WIND.)

5. CUT DOWN YOUR FAT INTAKE. DRINK SKIMMED OR SEMISKIMMED MILK. IF YOU EAT MEAT CHOOSE LEAN CUTS. USE LOWFAT SPREADS INSTEAD OF BUTTER.

6. TRY TO DO MORE EXERCISE. WALK, SWIM, CYCLE OR WORK OUT IN THE GYM.

7. WARMTH IS AN EXCELLENT REMEDY. IF YOU GET A PAINFUL TUMMY WRAP A HOT WATER BOTTLE IN A TOWEL AND HUG IT.

8. SPEND A LITTLE TIME LEARNING TO RELAX

9. INCREASE YOUR INTAKE OF FLUIDS – PARTICULARLY WATER.

10. DON'T DRINK TOO MUCH MILK. QUITE A LOT OF PEOPLE WHO SUFFER FROM IRRITABLE BOWEL SYNDROME REACT BADLY TO DAIRY FOODS.

ENDOMETRIOSIS

Each month the cells which make up the lining of the womb build up under hormonal control. Then, if no egg is fertilized, the lining breaks down and the discharge of the cells from the womb produces a monthly bleeding, or monthly period.

Problems can occur if the endometrial tissue is present outside the womb. If, for example, endometrial tissue is attached to the outer sides of the womb, or is wrapped around one of the ovaries then that tissue will respond to the monthly build up of hormones in exactly the same way as the endometrial tissue inside the womb. The cells will get thicker and thicker and eventually they will break down and bleed.

Inside the womb bleeding isn't really a problem. The blood is simply discharged through the vagina. But when the endometrial tissue is inside the abdominal cavity the blood cannot escape and there is often a considerable amount of pain. The pain of endometriosis can include backache.

The best way to treat endometriosis is often with hormones, but in some women surgery may be needed.

PROLAPSED WOMB

Normally, the womb or uterus sits in the abdomen with only the cervix projecting down into the vagina. The womb is kept in position by a network of muscles and ligaments. If these supports become weakened for any reason – and having lots of children is the most common cause – then the womb may fall down into the vagina.

Apart from childbirth other contributory factors include the menopause (which results in hormonal changes), obesity (which puts a straightforward physical strain on the tissues of the womb), heavy lifting (which can strain and weaken the muscles if not done properly), and violent coughing or sneezing (which increases the pressure inside the abdomen and helps to push the uterus out of the vagina).

Backache is a common symptom of a prolapse. If the prolapse is slight special pelvic floor muscle exercises may help. Alternatively a ring pessary – designed to hold the womb in position – may be the answer. However, if the prolapse is severe an operation may be needed to repair the tissues.

KIDNEY PROBLEMS

Kidney stones can cause a severe colicky pain in the lower back that comes and goes, while a kidney infection can cause a back pain that is both severe and constant. In the case of an infection there are usually other symptoms – such as a fever and/or bloodstained urine. The passing of urine may be painful too. Kidney problems need immediate medical attention. If there is an infection you will probably be given an antibiotic; if you have a kidney stone you may be taken into hospital in the hope that the stone will pass through by itself. In either case you will probably be advised by your doctor to drink plenty of fluids.

INDIGESTION AND STOMACH ULCER

Although the pain of indigestion and stomach ulceration usually affects the central part of the upper abdomen it may also develop in the middle of your back. This sort of pain is usually worst after a fatty, spicy or indigestible meal. If your doctor suspects that you have a problem of this type he should be able to prescribe effective medication and recommend changes to your daily lifestyle. For example, if you suffer from indigestion or stomach ulceration you may need to alter your diet and reduce your exposure to stress. You may also need to cut down your consumption of tobacco and/or alcohol.

OTHER POSSIBLE CAUSES

There are, of course, many other possible causes of back pain. Pneumonia, heart disease, gall stones, pancreatitis and shingles can all cause pain in the back in some patients. And although cancer of the spine itself is rare it is possible for cancers in other parts of the body to spread into the spine – damaging the bones and producing backache.

DEGENERATIVE CHANGE

Degenerative change is also the cause of much backache. Increasing age affects all the joints in your spine equally, but sometimes individual joints can start to break up far earlier than others – and degenerative changes can occur while you are still in your teens, though they are usually confined to only one or two joints.

GROWING OLD
CAN WEAKEN YOUR BACK

Although your back is designed to last you a lifetime it will get weaker as you get older – and the weaker it gets the more vulnerable it will become to damage and the less resistant it will be to stresses and strains. Gradually, your spine will become stiffer and the discs between your vertebrae will become less efficient as the body's natural shock absorbers.

The ageing process starts early in man – by the time you are about to leave your teens much of your body will be past its best – but many things accelerate the rate at which things are likely to go wrong.

If you put your spine under unusual amounts of pressure – either at work or on the sports field – you will almost certainly cause small amounts of damage to the discs, bones and ligaments of your back, and gradually over the years those small amounts of damage will build up. At the time that each injury occurs you may feel nothing more than a passing ache or pain, but over

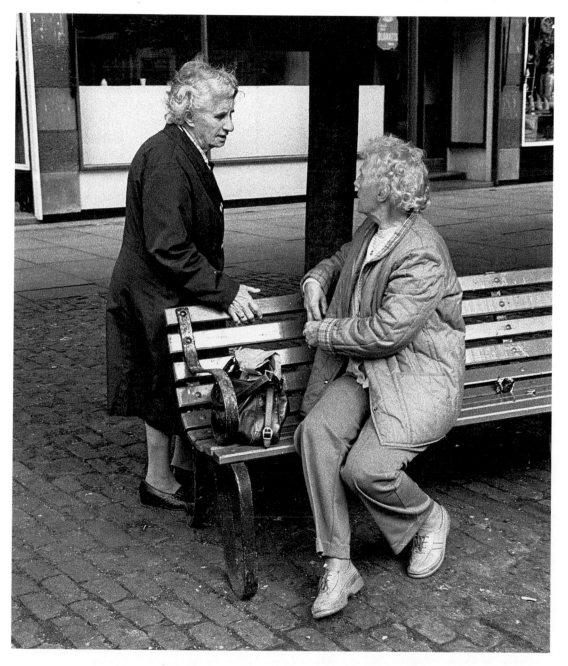

the years the damage may be more permanent.

You may also damage your spine if you sit or stand badly because your posture is poor.

DEGENERATION OF THE DISC

An intervertebral disc which has started to degenerate will be much thinner than normal, and although it won't be possible to see the change to the disc on an X-ray, it should be possible to make the diagnosis since the reduction in the size of the space will mean that the two vertebrae on either side of the disc will be closer together than usual.

In addition to being flatter and thinner the disc which has degenerated will also gradually become stiff and far tougher.

Disc problems usually develop fairly early in the degenerative process, since at this stage the disc is thinner and weaker than usual but has not yet become stiff, fibrous and tough. As a result of its weakness the disc will be far more likely to rupture – allowing the inner part to bulge outwards, causing nerve troubles and considerable amounts of pain.

The weakness of the disc will also mean that the surrounding joints and ligaments will be under far greater strain and consequently far more likely to collapse.

DEGENERATION OF THE JOINT

If the joints of your spine have to put up with abnormal amounts of wear and tear (as they will if you have to do a lot of straining, pushing, pulling and lifting, and you do not do all these things carefully) the cartilage lining your joints will become worn and thick, and the spaces through which your nerves have to pass will inevitably be reduced. The danger then is that back pains will develop – and won't go away. Sometimes the pains may not be obviously due to problems in your spine. For example, if the sciatic nerve is squeezed the resultant pain may affect the back of your leg.

DEGENERATION OF THE LIGAMENTS

If you hardly ever stretch your spine the ligaments between your vertebrae may become stiff, thin, inelastic, tender and painful. Inevitably, the stiffer your ligaments become the more stiff your spine will become, thus the less you will move and the more your ligaments will degenerate.

HOW YOUR BACK CAN BE INJURED

Your back is beautifully designed – and built to last. Neither bones nor muscles are likely to wear out even though they never stop moving. Every time you breathe your thoracic vertebrae (which are attached to your rib cage) will move. Every time you walk, sit down or stand up your back muscles and vertebrae will be moving. Even when you are asleep the bones and muscles of your back will be moving and vulnerable to stress and pressure. Your back is strong and capable and looked after properly it should last you a lifetime. Unfortunately, however, most backs do not get looked after properly. Occasionally, the damage is done suddenly – in an accident, for example – but, more commonly, the damage is done slowly over a long period of time, with a series of small mishaps responsible for the ensuing pain and misery. Most cases of backache are caused by a failure to understand how the back operates and many could undoubtedly be avoided with some thought and consideration.

Some of the ways in which you can inflict damage to the bones, muscles, ligaments and joints of your back are listed below.

BY SIMPLY STANDING

The human body was not designed to stand upright. When you do stand up gravity puts a tremendous stress on your whole spine. The bones at the bottom of your spine have to support the weight of all those bones above them. The pressure is far less damaging when you lie down or when you crawl about on all fours, though standing is better for you than sitting – particularly if you sit slumped in a soft chair.

BY MOVING ABOUT

Every time you move your spine will be jiggled and joggled about in a dozen different directions. Running – especially on hard surfaces – means thousands of vibrations, while even sitting in an apparently comfortable car, coach or train means that your spine will be subjected to an endless variety of vibrations. In order to protect the delicate spinal cord the bones, muscles and joints of your spine have to be able to absorb all these different pressures.

BY LIFTING THINGS

When you pick up something the pressure on your back goes up dramatically. If you lift something when your back is in a difficult or vulnerable position then you will be more prone to injury.

BY WEIGHING TOO MUCH

If you are overweight your spine will be under constant and unnecessary pressure. Women who are pregnant also put an extra strain on their backs – particularly towards the end of their pregnancies when they are at their heaviest.

BY TWISTING SUDDENLY

If you twist suddenly or unexpectedly the small muscles which hold your vertebrae in position can easily get torn. You may also injure one or more of your intervertebral discs. If the tear is a bad one then the fibrous outer-casing of an intervertebral disc may be weakened, with the result that the disc bulges outwards and you suffer pain. If the tear is a really bad one then the inside of the disc may be squeezed out through the gap in the outer casing.

BY JUMPING FROM A GREAT HEIGHT

When you jump from a modest height the discs in between your vertebrae absorb the force of your landing. But when you jump from a great height and land with a sudden crash, the discs may not be strong enough to absorb the shock wave which is transmitted through your feet, up your legs and into your spine. When that happens you may well fracture one of your vertebrae – either breaking off a piece of bone or shattering it completely. If the bone damages the spinal cord serious paralysis can result.

BY HAVING BAD POSTURE

If you stand or sit 'badly' then your whole spine will be thrown out of alignment and gradually, often over a period of years, you will develop more and more back problems. Wear and tear will be uneven and as muscles, joints and bones become unequally weak the stresses and strains on the other muscles, joints and bones in the rest of the body will increase – simply making things worse and worse.

BY EXERCISING UNWISELY

If you perform regular exercises which are not well designed and which put a strain on your spine you may create massive long-term problems for yourself. Some exercises – for example, those which involve incessant jumping up and down on hard floors – result in thousands of shock waves travelling up the spine. It is hardly surprising that injuries result. Other exercises involve putting unusually heavy strains on the spine when it is bent – once again injuries will be likely.

BY EXERCISING WITHOUT WARMING UP

If you suddenly start to exercise 'cold' untrained and weakened muscles you can easily strain them – particularly if you fail to 'warm up' properly. Common causes of back injury include attending a gym or digging the vegetable patch after years of inactivity, sweeping the drive clear of snow or leaves when the last exercise you had was months before, or finding an old tennis or squash racket and playing an energetic game without any preparation.

BY USING BADLY-DESIGNED EQUIPMENT

Much equipment in the home, office, car and factory may look good but be poorly designed in ergonomic terms. Desks and chairs are the worst offenders. Many people with back trouble can blame the fact that they have spent hours every day sitting on badly-designed chairs and working at a height that may have felt all right but that placed a constant strain on muscles, joints and bones.

BY WORRYING

Stress, pressure and anxiety can all cause muscle tension, especially in the back and shoulders, and tense muscles can cause pain and poor posture, and place unnecessary strains on bones and joints.

CHAPTER TWO

Slipped Discs

One of the most common problems to affect the back occurs when the nucleus pulposus – the soft, squashy part in the middle of the disc – bulges out through the tough, fibrous outer part of the disc and presses on whatever nerve or part of the spinal cord happens to be nearby.

The pain this can cause is often excruciating. If you've ever knocked your elbow – where the nerve runs across the surface of the bone and is easily trapped – you'll know just how painful a nerve injury can be.

"If you've ever knocked your elbow – where the nerve runs across the surface of the bone and is easily trapped – you'll know just how painful a nerve injury can be."

A disc prolapse – often but inaccurately called a 'slipped' disc – usually develops gradually as the disc degenerates with age.

However, the problem can be accelerated by a fall or a sudden, unexpected movement, and prolapsed discs can occur in younger people who take part in very strenuous activities – dancing and sport are common causes, as is sex.

It is usually people between their thirties and forties - who often think of themselves as being healthy - who are most likely to suffer from a prolapsed disc.

After the age of 30 the discs start to dehydrate and become slightly less pliable and this is when they are vulnerable.

But after another ten years or so the fibrous capsule around the outside of the disc becomes stiffer and stronger and the nucleus loses much of its moisture and shrinks considerably, making a prolapse less likely.

You may find your back getting slightly stiffer and less pliable as you get older and your in-built shock absorbers may be clearly slightly worn out, but there is a silver lining – you will be less likely to suffer from a prolapsed disc!

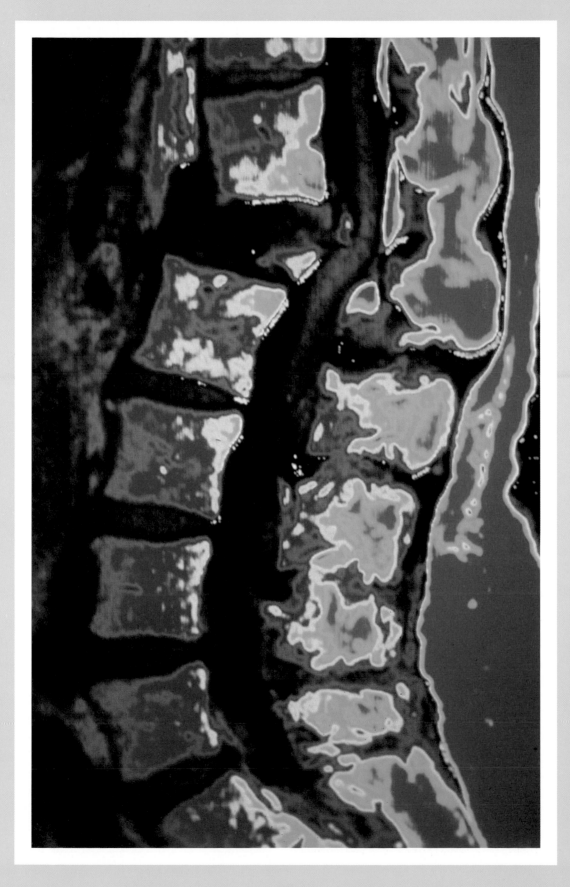

Disc problems are also slightly more common in men than in women – and they are particularly likely to affect individuals whose lifestyle is largely sedentary. They often develop after an unusually strenuous movement – for example, many people who suffer from disc protrusions will admit that they had noticed a pain after moving some furniture, digging in the garden,

able than discs elsewhere because it is here that the spine moves most – and is under most potential strain when you are lifting, pushing or pulling. The prolapse is usually backwards and sideways and the pain usually develops over a period of a day or so as the inflammation builds up and spreads. The resulting low back pain is then frequently accompanied by pain in the legs as

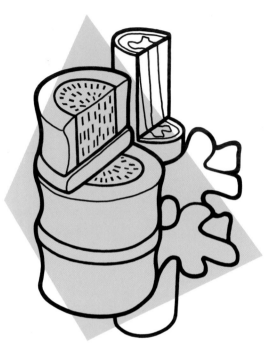

Normal disc between lumbar vertebrae

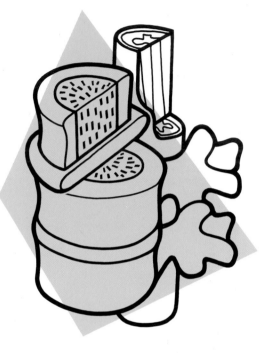

'Slipped' disc pressing on spinal cord

turning to pick something up out of the back of the car, or playing with a child or pet. There will have been a sharp twinge of pain, some stiffness and then – after a delay of a few hours or a day or so – a terrible pain and an inability to move.

In order to protect your spine – and reduce your chances of having a prolapsed disc – you need to exercise regularly to build up the flexibility of your spine and the strength of the muscles which hold its various parts in place.

Although disc prolapses can occur anywhere in the spine they most commonly occur at the bottom – in the lumbar region. The two discs that are most affected are the one between the fourth and fifth lumbar vertebrae and the one between the fifth lumbar vertebra and the top of the sacrum. These are probably more vulner-

the nerves which supply the leg muscles are affected.

In the condition known as 'sciatica', for example, the sciatic nerve – which supplies the hamstrings and other leg muscles – is affected. It is usual for the pain to be restricted to one side of the body – according to the direction of the protrusion. If a disc between the fourth and fifth lumbar vertebrae has been squeezed out to the right then the right leg will be affected. In addition to pain, a nerve that is being 'pinched' may also produce a wide variety of other sensations – with numbness and 'pins and needles' being among the most common.

In those relatively rare conditions where the disc protrusion occurs higher up the spine the area affected by pain will again depend upon the position of the protrusion. If a disc has prolapsed in the neck then the shoulder and arm and head will be affected. If a disc has prolapsed in the middle of the back (and this is the most uncommon place of all because the middle of the back is relatively immobile) then the trunk may be the only part of the body that suffers.

Because the discs themselves have virtually no nerve supply it is only when a disc prolapses and presses onto a nerve or some other vulnerable part of your spine that you will notice any symptoms. The pain of a prolapsed disc tends to be deep, dull and persistent and it may radiate into all sorts of unexpected places. For example, a prolapsed disc in the lower back may produce pain in several places such as the buttocks, hip or groin. Some people find that these pains are worse if they bend in one particular way. Others find that their pains become unbearable if they stand up straight. And it isn't uncommon for people to complain that their pain is worse when they sneeze, cough or laugh.

If you have a slipped disc the first thing your doctor will want to do will be to make sure that your problem *is* caused by a disc that is misbehaving – and if it is a disc that is causing the trouble he or she will want to know which one.

If there is then any doubt, to investigate your back problem an orthopaedic surgeon (who specializes in bone problems) and/or a neurosurgeon (who specializes in nerve troubles) will probably want to perform a number of investigations and tests: X-rays, CT scans, myelography (in which a radio-opaque substance is injected around the spinal cord) and discography (in which a radio-opaque substance is injected directly into the disc itself so that it can be seen clearly on an X-ray).

In addition tests of electrical activity in the muscles may be done to see which muscles are being affected.

Disc problems respond well to bed rest (though you may have to experiment to find the best and most comfortable position in bed), and although a protruding disc may return to its normal position spontaneously in a few days you may need to stay in bed for several weeks. The length of time you'll need to rest will depend partly on the position of the protrusion and its size, and partly on how your body has responded to the pain. If your muscles have become very tense as a result of the pain you may find it difficult to move at all even though the disc has returned to its original position. You must have a firm mattress and it is important that you stay where your are for as long as the disc is out of position – getting up and moving about will usually make things worse, because when you are standing the weight of the upper part of your body will press down on the disc, making it impossible for the protruded piece of disc to get back into its proper position thus increasing the pressure on any nerve that is being squashed.

Roughly half of all sufferers will get better within a month – with quite a number of those making a full recovery within two weeks – and nine out of ten sufferers from 'slipped' discs will have made a fairly full recovery within six weeks, whatever treatment they have. A small number of sufferers are left with a tiny patch of numbness or some muscle weakness, but most are so relieved that the main pains have gone that they don't mind too much about these.

Apart from bed rest there are lots of things that you can do to help yourself and your doctor will undoubtedly also help by telling you which treatments you should try. Mobilizing exercises will probably be vital as you begin to recover and you may find the manipulation from an osteopath or chiropractor will reduce the pain and improve your ability to get around. Acupuncture, which helps to relieve pain and to relax muscles, can be extremely effective.

Doctors can, of course, prescribe painkillers to deaden the pain, though it is vitally important that you take pills properly. (There is an important section on drugs for pain relief on page 70.) When you start to get up out of bed and move around you may be advised to wear a special corset to support your spine – many people find that a corset doesn't just relieve the pain but also increases their confidence.

If, after a decent period of rest and treatment (six weeks or so is the usually accepted interval), the pain is still there then your doctors will – probably with some reluctance – start to think about surgery. (See page 72.) Back surgery is never easy, and wise surgeons don't rush patients into the operating theatre unnecessarily because there is always a risk that things may be made worse. If surgery is contemplated then your doctors will want to do whatever tests have not yet been done in order to find out exactly where the problem lies and how severe it is.

WHEN A PROLAPSED DISC STAYS OUT

If a disc prolapse does not go back, but stays out of position, it can cause chronic long–term pain. The nature and extent of the pain will, of course, depend on the position of the prolapse and the nerve that is being compressed. The biggest danger is that if a nerve remains pinched for a long period of time then it may be permanently damaged – with the result that the muscles which are normally controlled by that nerve will become weak and ineffective.

If a disc in the lumbar spine stays prolapsed then you will probably feel a constant aching and stiffness in your back – particularly if you have been sitting down or stuck in any one position for a long period of time. The back pain will probably be on one side of your body and may be accompanied by pains in your leg or by 'pins and needles' in your leg.

You will also probably find that any heavy lifting or indeed anything that puts a strain on your back will lead to a worsening of the pain.

If the basic problem is in your neck then the general symptoms will be similar. In addition to generalized aching you may also notice occasional nerve pains, and sudden twisting or turning will probably make things worse – and may bring on a particularly painful episode. You may also discover some fairly unpleasant sounding grinding noises in your neck because of the strain on the ligaments and joints. People with neck problems invariably find that stress, tension, anxiety and pressure all make things considerably worse – and, indeed, the severest problems may coincide with the moments of greatest tension at work or at home.

Wherever in your spine lies the problem you will find that to build up your resistance to pain you will need to exercise regularly. This will help to build up the strength of the muscles around your spine and to reduce the stress on the bones, ligaments and joints of your spine.

You may also benefit from manipulation and acupuncture, and you will almost certainly benefit if you learn to relax yourself thoroughly as often as possible.The good news is that as you get older your spine will gradually stiffen and your ligaments will become tougher. As this happens so the pain should reduce.

TESTS YOUR DOCTOR MAY DO

X-RAYS

Discs, being soft tissues, do not show up on X-rays, but it is often possible to spot disc damage by looking at the size of the spaces between the vertebrae. A narrowed disc will show up on an X-ray as bony vertebrae being closer together than normal. Most of the time, however, X-rays merely exclude more serious damage and do not show up anything useful. In at least 90 per cent of patients X-rays do not provide any positive diagnostic information.

DISCOGRAPHY

In this procedure a contrast medium which will be visible on X-rays will be injected directly into one of your intervertebral discs. You will be given a local anaesthetic and then, with a long thin needle, a doctor will inject the contrast medium directly into your disc. X-ray pictures will then be taken to determine where the problem is. There may be some soreness at the site of the injection. The X-rays will show a rough outline of the disc, and if the outer part of the disc has ruptured then the contrast medium will leak out and be visible outside the disc.

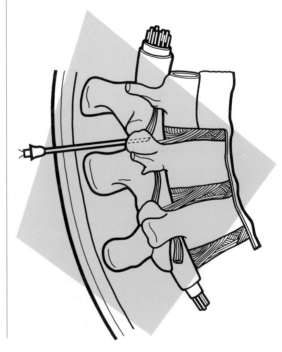

MYELOGRAPHY

In order to perform a myelogram doctors inject a radio-opaque dye into your spinal canal and then take X-ray pictures of the dye. Using a local anaesthetic the doctors will make a small hole directly into your spine so that they can inject the dye into the tiny space around the spinal cord and the nerves which come from it. The operation will be done on a table which tilts so that the doctors can move you up and down to make the dye run up and down your spine and around various different nerve junctions. The whole procedure lasts around half an hour. This is an unpleasant, tricky and potentially hazardous procedure, and you will

Diagnosing a back problem

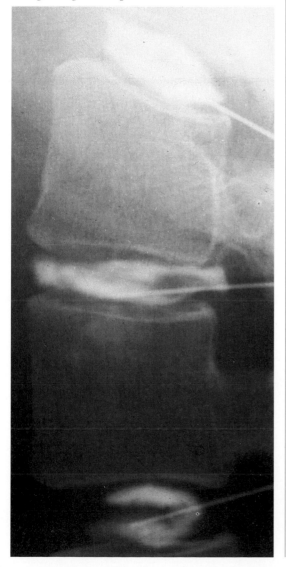

usually need to spend a day in hospital if you are having this test. The side effects – which seem to affect quite a number of patients having this test – include headache, nausea and vomiting. In the past some patients are believed to have suffered long–term problems as a result of damage – arachnoiditis – done by an oil–based dye, and so today most doctors use a water–soluble contrast material. Because of the dangers associated with this procedure it is usually only performed when a surgeon intends to operate and wants an accurate idea of the sort of damage that may exist in the spine.

CT SCAN

Computerized tomography is painless and fairly fast. It uses a very sophisticated computer–operated X-ray machine which takes a series of pictures throughout the spine and produces a three–dimensional view of any damage that exists. Unlike an ordinary X-ray a scanner does not just show bones but also soft tissues like muscles. A scanner will probably help your doctor look at your vertebrae and discs to form a diagnosis more accurately than anything else.

ELECTROMYOGRAPHY

By inserting fine needles into your muscles and measuring the electrical impulses, electromyography enables doctors to measure the activity of various muscles – and it therefore helps them to decide which nerves have been damaged. (When a nerve has been damaged the muscles normally associated with that nerve will be less active than usual.) Electromyography takes about half an hour and is fairly painless and free of side effects.

SURGERY – A DECOMPRESSION OPERATION

If you have symptoms of a prolapsed disc which persist and which include chronic, intractable and untreatable pain then a surgeon may be asked to consider whether or not a decompression operation might help. Before doing an operation a surgeon will almost certainly want to perform at least one (and probably more) of the investigations described above. The decompression operation is described on page 72.

CHAPTER THREE

How To Keep Your Back Healthy

Whether you suffer from backache or simply want to keep your healthy back in form you should read this chapter carefully. It will tell you how to prevent backache developing, how you can maintain your back in good condition and how you can avoid back trouble in the future.

Remember that at least eight out of ten cases of backache are caused by muscle tension – usually produced by poor posture, stress or carelessness. Thus *in eight out of ten cases backache can be avoided.*

> *"When you're lifting or picking things up you should take care not to bend from the waist. You should bend at the knees and keep your back as straight as possible."*

The first thing you *must* remember is that lifting or carrying heavy loads is one of the most common causes of back trouble. According to a series of studies conducted by Surrey University approximately 20,000 nurses working in Britain's National Health Service suffer from back pain every year and most of them get their pain because they have lifted or moved heavy patients.

When you're lifting or picking things up you should take care not to bend from the waist. You should bend at the knees and keep your back as straight as possible. It may feel natural to lift by bending your back and reaching down, but doing so puts a tremendous amount of strain on your back muscles.

Here are some more tips to avoid straining your back muscles. Firstly make sure that your bed is not contributing to your problem. A firm mattress will keep your back in good condition; if your mattress is saggy put a board under it to make it firmer. You should sleep on your side with your knees bent slightly, sleeping on your stomach increases the likelihood of back pain developing.

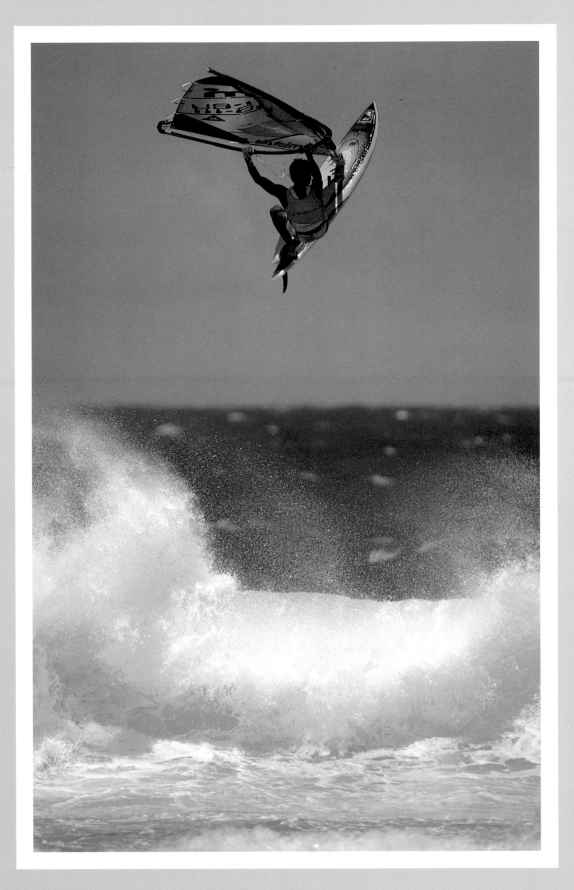

Secondly, avoid high-heeled shoes whenever possible. They throw the spine out of line and can lead to long-term pain problems.

Be careful how you sit. If you spend a lot of time sitting and working at a desk do make sure that your desk and chair are at the correct relative working heights. Sit with your back straight and make sure that your desk is well lit, and do get up and stretch your back muscles regularly.

If you are doing paperwork it is best to rest books and papers that you are reading on a stand so that you don't have to lean over.

In a car adjust the seat regularly – car seats are notoriously troublesome. Put a cushion at the base of your spine. On long journeys it is especially important that you stop your car regularly and go for a walk round for a few minutes. Do a few stretching and bending exercises too – they will really help you.

Prolonged standing in one position will put a tremendous strain on your back. Remember to stand up straight and pull in your abdomen, and don't stand for long periods – sit down occasionally. If you're at a party keep circulating around the room, and, if you're drinking at a bar lean first on one elbow and then on the other elbow.

This may sound slightly trivial, but heavy shoulder-bags are bad for your spine unless you move them from one side to the other at regular intervals.

Another tip is to lose any excess weight. If you are overweight you *must* diet. I can't stress too much how important that is. Ten pounds – just ten pounds – of excess weight carried on your abdomen is equivalent to a pressure of 100 pounds of additional weight inside your spine. So just imagine how much damage 40 or 50 extra pounds of fat can do. As your abdomen get bigger so your buttocks are pushed out to balance the weight increase, and so your spine gets pushed out of shape too. All this explains why back pain is so common among pregnant women.

Finally, I think it's well worth pointing out that exercise – done regularly and gently – will help to strengthen your back and tone up your muscles. Swimming and walking are probably two of the best forms of exercise – both will help to build up your back muscles and keep your ligaments in good condition.

TEN TIPS FOR LIFTING WITHOUT DAMAGING YOUR BACK

LIFTING HEAVY OBJECTS IS A MAJOR CAUSE OF BACK TROUBLE. FOLLOW THESE TIPS TO HELP PROTECT YOUR BACK:

1. THERE IS NO ACCEPTABLE DEFINITION OF HEAVY. ANY LOAD CAN DAMAGE YOUR BACK IF YOU LIFT WRONGLY. ALWAYS LIFT CAREFULLY AND ALWAYS THINK BEFORE LIFTING.

2. WHENEVER POSSIBLE WORK OUT A WAY TO MINIMIZE THE EFFORT REQUIRED. IF THERE IS A MECHANICAL HOIST AVAILABLE – USE IT. IF YOU CAN USE A TROLLEY OR BARROW THEN USE ONE. UNLOAD CUPBOARDS AND TAKE HEAVY FURNITURE APART WHENEVER POSSIBLE. IF THERE IS NOTHING ON THE OBJECT TO HOLD ONTO, THEN USE A SLING OR PUT A STRONG ROPE UNDERNEATH IT. IF THERE IS HELP AVAILABLE WAIT UNTIL IT ARRIVES. PLAN TO LIFT AND MOVE HEAVY OBJECTS IN GENTLE, EASY STAGES. STOP IF YOU FEEL TIRED – THAT IS WHEN ACCIDENTS HAPPEN.

3. IF YOU HAVE TO MOVE A HEAVY WEIGHT ON A TROLLEY REMEMBER THAT PULLING USUALLY PUTS LESS STRAIN ON YOUR BODY THAN PUSHING.

4. MAKE SURE THAT YOU WEAR SHOES WITH NON-SLIP SOLES. DO NOT TRY LIFTING OR CARRYING HEAVY WEIGHTS WHILE WEARING HIGH HEELS. IF POSSIBLE WEAR SHOES THAT PROVIDE

PROPER PROTECTION IN CASE SOMETHING HEAVY DROPS ON YOUR FEET. AND MAKE SURE THAT YOU USE GLOVES WITH A GOOD GRIP. DON'T TRY LIFTING IN UNUSUALLY LOOSE OR TIGHT CLOTHING, IN CLOTHING THAT RESTRICTS YOUR MOVEMENTS IN ANY WAY OR IN CLOTHING THAT MIGHT 'CATCH' ON A PROTRUSION.

5. STAND CLOSE TO THE OBJECT YOU WANT TO LIFT WITH YOUR FEET APART TO IMPROVE YOUR BALANCE. PUT ONE FOOT SLIGHTLY AHEAD OF THE OTHER.

6. BEND YOUR HIPS AND YOUR KNEES AND KEEP YOUR BACK STRAIGHT AND YOUR SHOULDERS LEVEL AND IN LINE WITH YOUR PELVIS. PICK UP THE OBJECT YOU ARE LIFTING WITH THE WHOLE OF YOUR HAND (RATHER THAN JUST YOUR FINGER TIPS) AND KEEP YOUR ARMS CLOSE IN TO YOUR BODY. A WEIGHT HELD OUT AT ARMS' LENGTH PUTS TEN TIMES THE STRAIN ON YOUR SPINE AS A WEIGHT HELD CLOSE TO YOUR BODY.

7. BRACE YOUR ABDOMINAL MUSCLES AND THEN LIFT THE OBJECT BY STRAIGHTENING YOUR KNEES. IF YOU ARE TRYING TO LIFT SOMETHING VERY HEAVY HALVE THE STRESS BY LIFTING ONE END FIRST. IF YOU HAVE TO TURN MOVE YOUR FEET AS WELL AS YOUR BODY AND DO NOT TWIST OR BEND YOUR BODY WHILE LIFTING.

8. TRY TO LIFT SMOOTHLY, AND REMEMBER TO KEEP THE OBJECT CLOSE TO YOUR BODY ALL THE TIME.

9. IF THE OBJECT IS TOO HEAVY FOR YOU PUT IT DOWN STRAIGHTAWAY.

10. WHEN PUTTING A LOAD DOWN LOWER YOURSELF BY BENDING YOUR KNEES AND SQUATTING. DO NOT BEND YOUR BACK – THIS IS WHEN INJURIES OFTEN HAPPEN.

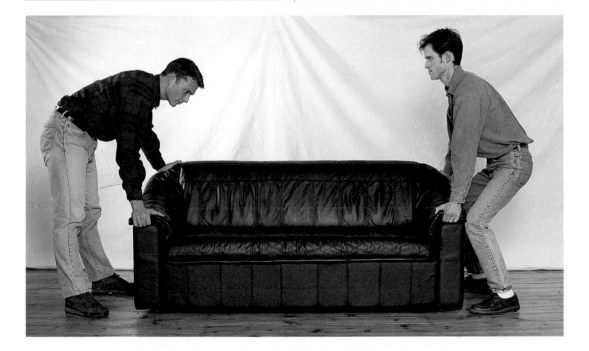

HOW TO SLEEP SAFELY

If you regularly wake up feeling stiff – and have to move around to get rid of that stiffness – then there is a good chance that your bed is damaging your back. Most of us spend one-third of our lives in our beds and benefit fully from sleep only if we are comfortable throughout the night. A good bed is vital.

WHAT SORT OF BED IS BEST?

A very soft bed which has a saggy mattress may seem comfortable when you first lie on it, but it will make your vertebral column sag during the night and that will stretch the ligaments which connect your bones. The result will be pain and stiffness.

To protect your back your bed should have a solid base with a firm mattress. Don't bother spending extra money on a special orthopaedic mattress – I don't think they are likely to be any better than an ordinary, firm mattress. In general it is probably better to buy a mattress that seems slightly too hard than one that seems slightly soft. Remember that after you have been lying on it for a few weeks your mattress will undoubtedly lose some of its rigidity. (Remember too that it is possible to have a bed that is *too* firm.)

When testing a mattress lie on it and try to slide your hand in between the small of your back and the top of the mattress. If there is an obvious gap then the mattress may well be too hard. If there is no gap and you cannot easily push your hand in between your back and the mattress then the bed will almost certainly be too soft. You should be able to roll from side to side on your mattress – if you cannot roll around on it but simply sink into a hollow created by your weight then the bed is too soft.

If you cannot afford a new bed and the bed you have has a soft or sagging base, you can make it firmer by putting a board between the base and the mattress. The board should be as wide as the bed base and should go down as far as your thighs. If you use a couple of old doors to add firmness to your bed do remember to take the handles off first!

If you and your partner are very different weights or have quite different requirements you may need to buy two single beds which can be linked together.

WHAT ABOUT PILLOWS?

Special pillows are not usually necessary. It is, however, sensible to make sure that you use the right number of pillows and of the correct consistency. A good pillow should be fairly firm (you should be able to balance it on your arm without the two ends flopping down on either side) and should keep your neck vertebrae in a straight line with the vertebrae in the rest of your spine. The best way to find the most suitable pillow for you is to experiment until you find something that enables you to wake up in the morning without suffering from an aching neck.

THE RIGHT BEDCLOTHES

You will find sleeping under a duvet much better than sheets and blankets for two main reasons. First, you will find it easier to get into and out of bed without straining your back if you sleep under a duvet. Second, and just as important, you will find it much easier to re-make your bed if you use a duvet than if you use sheets and blankets.

If, however, you do use sheets and blankets, kneel down to tuck in sheets. Do not bend over the bed with your back arched – if you do you'll quickly end up with a sore and painful back.

HOW TO GET IN AND OUT OF BED

A remarkable number of people injure their backs clambering into and out of bed.

When getting into bed you should sit down on the edge of the mattress and then lower your body onto your side while bending your knees and lifting your feet up onto the bed.

When getting out of bed you should bend your knees up, roll onto your side (if you aren't already) and then push yourself up into a sitting position allowing your legs to swing slowly out of bed.

HOW TO TACKLE YOUR WEIGHT PROBLEM SUCCESSFULLY

Excess weight caused by overeating is one of the most common causes of backache, and it is, of course, a common cause of many other disorders too. If you weigh too much you are also more likely to develop heart disease, get high blood pressure, have a stroke or suffer from diabetes.

Although it is impossible to know exactly how many people die due to being overweight my guess is that unwanted fat kills millions of people a year. In addition, excess fat makes many lives miserable, causes depression and makes crippling diseases such as asthma and arthritis considerably worse.

Heart disease of all kinds is intensified when patients weigh too much. In many cases heart disease is brought on because of obesity. The fatter you are the greater the burden will be on your heart. Every year millions of people die prematurely of heart disease. Thousands of those are in their thirties and forties, and many are overweight.

Diabetes mellitus is now so common that 2 per cent of the population have it, and the number of diabetics is doubling every ten years. Many patients become diabetic because they eat too much. Thousands of cases of diabetes could be prevented if people ate less fattening food.

Eczema, varicose veins, piles, high blood pressure, gall stones, strokes, hernias – the list of disorders made worse by overweight is virtually endless. Yet despite all these problems and all this misery no one in the medical profession seems to take obesity seriously!

Doctors are generally unsympathetic when asked for slimming advice. One recent major survey showed that over half of would-be dieters said that it was a waste of time visiting a doctor to ask for slimming advice. Another big survey showed that almost one-third of family doctors are themselves *fat*. The advice given most often to overweight patients is simply an unhelpful: 'eat less'.

When did you last see a Government poster or TV advertisement warning of the dangers of obesity? Governments spend a fortune warning us of the hazards of relatively rare problems but virtually nothing on being overweight – the biggest health problem in the Western world – and one that kills thousands who could so easily be saved.

TV producers seem to regard being overweight as a trivial subject, suitable only for afternoon programmes aimed at women. I've lost count of the number of pro-

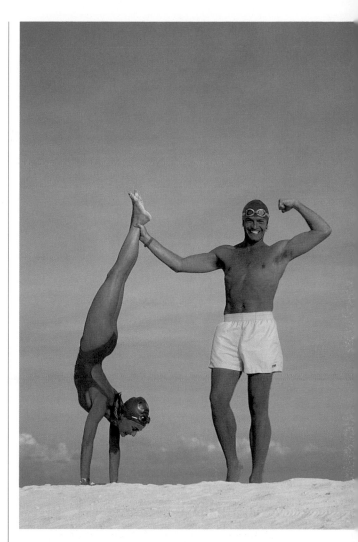

grammes that have been made showing us 97 ways to stuff a turkey and there have been dozens of problems dealing with drug addiction. But I can't remember ever seeing a TV programme asking *why* obesity is so commonplace or *what* can be done about it. Food programmes pontificate endlessly about the merits of the wok but never seem concerned about the fact that their chubby presenters are simply encouraging more and more overeating.

Indeed, virtually the only coverage dieting seems to get comes when people overdo it. Every time an anorexia victim tells her story in public the blame inevitably falls on slimming magazines and organizations which are trying to help people lose weight.

The truth is that the majority of fat people *want* to lose their excess weight. They *want* to look more attractive. They *want* to feel fitter and healthier. The truth is that obesity is unnatural and unhealthy. It is a consequence of a mixture of bad habits, over-indulgence and commercially inspired greed.

So, here's how you can lose weight – permanently. Forget all the unsuccessful diets you've tried in the past. You *can* lose weight successfully without going on a special diet, without having to avoid every food that you like, without feeling hungry all the time, without living on a diet of lettuce, cucumber and tomatoes, and

I get fat in the first place? People get fat for all sorts of different reasons but three of the most important are boredom, guilt and depression. Individually, these are undoubtedly the three most dangerous enemies any slimmer has. Together they can combine to destroy the most carefully planned dietary programme.

They *can* be overcome – as long as you understand how these forces develop, how they can affect your life and what you can do to protect yourself.

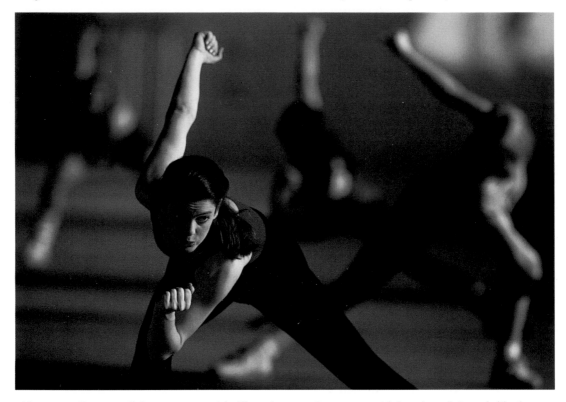

without spending a small fortune on special pills and food supplements.

First, of course, you have got to really *want* to lose weight. And you've got to know *why* you want to lose weight. Any diet started without incentive or determination will be doomed to failure.

If you lose weight you will be healthier, feel fitter and stronger, and look better. You'll gain confidence and self-assurance and you'll be more at ease with your body. Most important of all, your back will be far less likely to cause you pain. Getting rid of your excess weight will probably help your back problem as much as anything else you can do and almost certainly *more* than anything your doctor can do.

The next question you must ask yourself is *why* did

Let us start with boredom. It is probably the most common and yet the most underestimated problem around these days. Whether you work as a housewife or you have a dull job in an office or a tedious one on a factory assembly line, boredom can result in your nibbling and bingeing without really being aware of what you are doing. The only real answer is to try and add a little more excitement to your life in as many ways as you possibly can.

Stop for a moment and try to think back to when you were much younger. Try to imagine the dreams you had; the things you wanted to do. Some of those dreams, some of the things you wanted to do when you were younger, are still possible. So, for example, if you have always wanted to paint or write, then why not start now? You can probably get all the advice and information you need at your public library and at evening classes at a local college.

It doesn't matter *what* you do, as long as you do something that adds excitement and zest to your life. Take up gardening if that is what you fancy – if you haven't got a garden, get an allotment somewhere locally or offer to help cultivate a neighbour's garden for a share of the produce. Learn about carpentry or take up car maintenance or flower arranging!

If you add new hobbies to your life you will benefit twice over. Firstly, you will enjoy the excitement and pleasure of your new hobby, and you won't be tempted into nibbling because you are bored. And secondly, as you build up your interest you will find that there won't be anywhere near as much time left for thinking about food.

Many people who have a weight problem become obsessed with the idea of food and find themselves thinking about it all day long – particularly when they are trying to diet. If you fill up your life with things that you enjoy doing you will beat that particular problem, because the best way to beat an obsession is not to tackle it head on but simply to put it into its rightful place.

Next, consider guilt – another powerful driving force and another reason why so many people are desperately overweight. Nearly all fat people suffer from guilt. They are kind, gentle, generous people who want to please everyone, and they suffer enormously because they find that they simply cannot do everything that everyone wants them to do. They feel guilty each time they have to let other people down.

On top of all that guilt there is feeling of the guilt about overeating. When you unwrap a packet of biscuits to cheer yourself up, and then munch your way through as many of them as you can, you feel guilty about being overweight because you feel that you are letting everyone down. All that guilt then produces shame, depression and a complete lack of self-confidence. Because they feel guilty about their eating habits thousands of slimmers like you feel inadequate and

"Boredom can result in your nibbling and binging without really being aware of what you are really doing."

unsuccessful. They consider themselves to be failures.

If you are going to overcome your guilt and your feelings of inadequacy and get rid of your view of yourself as a failure, then you need to build up your self-esteem and give yourself more confidence.

Start by thinking of all your virtues. Pretend you are writing an advertisement for yourself and write down everything complimentary that you can. If you are always punctual put that down. If you are neat add that to your list. If you are kind to animals, thoughtful with old people and gentle with children, add those. Make a note of your physical strengths as well as your mental strengths, social virtues and other good points. Finally, write down all the times when you can remember having succeeded in avoiding the temptation to overeat. Try to remember all the times when you've said 'no' when you have been tempted to say 'yes' instead.

The more you can build up your own image of yourself as a success – rather than as a failure – the stronger you will be the next time temptation comes your way.

Next, you must learn to deal with unhappiness, disappointment and depression without using food to cheer yourself up. You probably got into the habit of doing that when you were small. Your mother may have given you some sweets when you were good; or you may have been sent to bed without any pudding when you were naughty. Either way you will have got into the habit of associating happiness with food. You must now break this link by learning to cheer yourself up in other ways.

If you are feeling miserable and tempted to start comfort eating go for a brisk walk around the building or beat the carpets. Pick up the telephone and ring a friend if you feel like breaking into the biscuit tin.

Boredom, guilt and unhappiness are among the most common reasons for diets failing. Once you have conquered these three destructive forces you will be far more able to stick to your dieting programme and lose your excess weight effectively.

The next step is to take complete responsibility for

what you eat and for your weight. Lots of overweight people blame other people for their weight problem. They blame people for forcing food on them. They blame their parents, husband, wife, children and friends. But you have to take responsibility onto your own shoulders. If you are going to deal with your weight problem effectively and permanently then you have to take back the responsibility for your own eating habits – otherwise there will always be an excuse.

The next important decision you have to take is: how much weight do you want to lose and in how long a period. Try to decide what weight you should be or what weight you will feel comfortable at, and then deduct that from your current weight. When you have decided how much weight you need to lose, my advice is that you should aim at losing two pounds a week. That is a good, attainable safe target. Two pounds a week may not sound very much but if you lose two pounds a week regularly then the weight loss will soon mount up. And if you plan your diet properly you will be able to keep your fat off for ever.

"The more you think of yourself as a failure the more you will fail. To succeed you have to think of yourself as a success."

To make things easier for yourself break up your overall target into a series of smaller targets. Pick a date in your diary just three or four weeks ahead and aim to have lost six or eight pounds by then. That is your immediate, short-term target. The extra beauty about having a short-term target is that every time you hit your target your confidence will soar and you will find that losing weight becomes easier and easier.

Confidence is really important for successful slimmers. You've got to get rid of that old 'I'm no good at dieting' image or that vision of yourself as the world's worst slimmer. The more you think of yourself as a failure the more you will fail. To succeed you have got to think of yourself as a success.

Well over 90 per cent of the people who try to lose weight – and who succeed in the short term – are overweight again within a few months. They invariably fail because they don't have the determination and confidence they need in order to succeed.

I am often asked to sum up the secret of successful slimming in a few words. It's easy. I can do it in one sentence: *'Eat when you are hungry – and stop eating when you are not hungry.'*

It sounds obvious, doesn't it? But I wonder how many times you have thought about losing weight in such simple terms?

The fact is that there is an appetite control centre in your brain which is designed to make sure that you eat exactly what your body needs – and when you need to eat it. If you have a fluctuating or recurring weight problem, then it is probable that you have been ignoring your appetite control centre and you are eating not according to your body's needs but according to outside influences dictated by the people around you.

If you have a long-lasting weight problem then the chances are high that your eating habits were established when you were young. Think back to when you were small and you may remember that you were always encouraged to eat at organized mealtimes. Your mother probably got upset when you didn't eat up everything on your plate. Those early behavioural patterns will have helped to ensure that your appetite control centre got consistently overruled.

The result is that your current eating habits are almost certainly controlled not by your body's genuine need for food but by a totally artificial idea of its requirements. You have got used to eating according to the clock on the wall rather than the clock in your brain. You eat what the advertising copywriters want you to eat, not what your body wants you to eat. And, just as important, you fail to stop eating when you are no longer hungry.

Fortunately, all those damaging eating habits can be reversed. If you learn to listen to your body's internal signs of hunger, learn to break life-long habits which overrule your appetite control centre and teach yourself to eat when you need to, then you will be able to get slim and stay slim.

The appetite control centre in your brain is controlled by the amount of sugar circulating in your blood, and it will tell you exactly when you need to eat

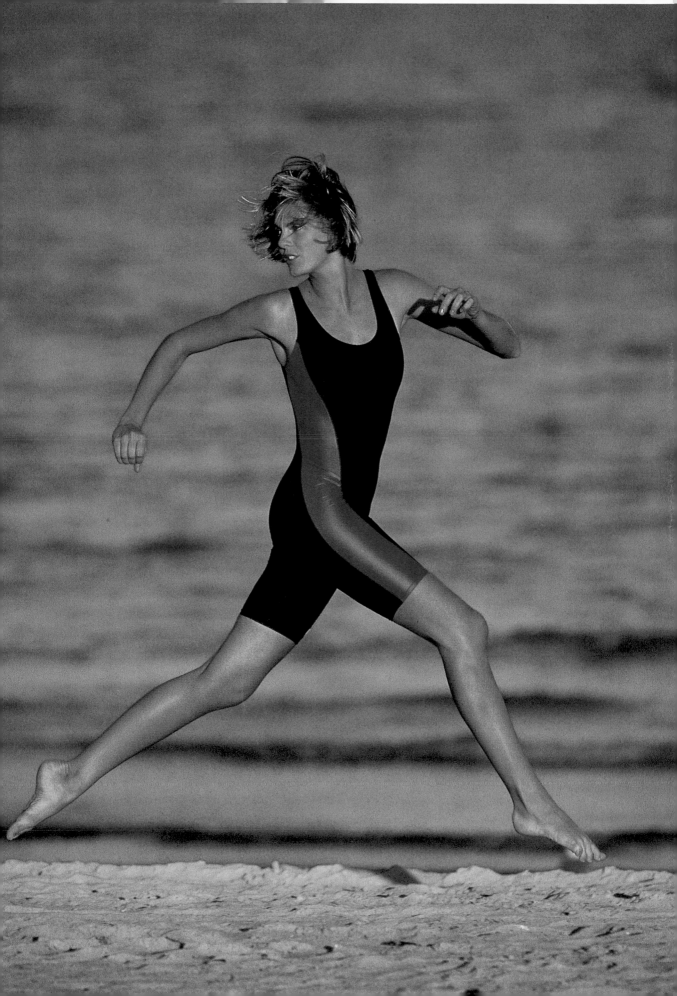

and how much you need. There is no doubt that if you can listen to your appetite control centre you will never overeat and therefore never get fat again.

Look around you next time you eat out and you will see that most people finish off everything on their plate – however much was put there in the first place. You may have also got into the habit of eating, almost without thinking, while reading, working or watching television. As a result you may often have little idea of what you are eating – or how much. You just carry on until you feel bloated or until everything has gone.

In order to lose your excess weight – and maintain your weight at the level you would like it to be – you must learn to use your intuition to help you tell when you are hungry and when you have had enough to eat. Try to get into the habit of eating not according to strict mealtimes but according to your natural needs. And, just as important, try to get into the habit of stopping eating when you are no longer hungry. Listen to your body. Don't wait until you are overfull.

You must also learn to be more assertive when you are eating. *You* must decide how much food you want to eat, and you must decide whether or not you have a second helping. Don't let other people push you around. Don't let other people make you feel guilty if you don't eat up everything they want you to eat. Remember it is *your* body.

To help yourself eat less than you really need – and therefore lose weight – you can trick your body by eating filling but low-calorie snacks when you feel hungry or just before you are about to have a meal. For example, if you have a cup of black coffee or lemon tea, a one-calorie soft drink or a bowl of clear soup half an hour before you have a meal you won't feel as hungry when you start eating. You will eat less than you would otherwise have done.

When you put food onto your plate spread it around to make it look as if there is a lot there. Pick a

"In order to lose your excess weight - and maintain your weight at the level you would like to be - you must learn to use your intuition to help you tell when you are hungry and when you have had enough to eat."

small plate, and choose foods such as raw or slightly cooked vegetables that need a lot of chewing, that will help to slow you down and make you feel as though you have had a good meal. Never be frightened to leave food on your plate when you are full, and if you consistently find that there is food left over try putting less on your plate to start with.

Don't eat huge meals at infrequent intervals just because that is the way you have been taught to eat. If you eat a meal and then don't eat for several hours your body will react accordingly. It will expect to receive supplies of food irregularly. Consequently, it will encourage you to eat as much as possible when you are eating so that it can then store up what isn't needed. The food that is stored up will end as fat deposits. If, on the other hand, you eat smaller meals more frequently, the food you take in will be burned up straight away. None of it will be stored and you will take in just what your body needs.

Remember to concentrate on what you are doing when you are eating. If you are doing something else – like reading or talking – then the chances are that you will miss the messages that your appetite control centre is trying to give you.

Try to build up an awareness of your body's needs. If you eat something salty you will feel thirsty afterwards because your body will try to balance the high salt intake with a higher fluid intake. Listen to your body when you are hungry and you will find that it is often telling you the truth about what you need to eat. If you really feel like something sweet then eat something sweet. If you have been ignoring your body for years it will take you a while to learn how to listen to it again – but if you persevere then you will succeed.

You now know the secrets of long–term slimming success, but you have to change the habits of a lifetime. I know that isn't easy so I have prepared a special short script that you can record and listen to everyday in order to boost your determination to succeed. Speak slowly while recording the tape.

Simply listen to it every morning and every evening for a week. It should take you no more than five minutes. After a week, if you are confident that you are winning your battle, you can listen to the tape just once a day – either first thing in the morning or last thing at night. I think you will find that the tape will be most effective if you listen to it through headphones fitted to a small personal stereo, and try to listen somewhere where you can be quiet and undisturbed.

THE SLIMMING TAPE SCRIPT

Before you start to listen to this tape make sure that you are really comfortable. Either sit yourself down in an easy chair or lie down on your bed. Try to make sure that no one will disturb you for a few minutes. Shut the door and take the telephone off the hook if necessary.

Now, close your eyes and take big, slow, deep breaths. Count up to four while you are breathing in. Then, hold your breath while you count up to two. Next, breathe out – again counting up to four as you do so. When you have emptied your lungs hold that position for another count of two and then start the whole process again by taking another deep breath. Breathing deeply will help you relax.

Try to relax your mind by conjuring up some restful and peaceful scene. Imagine, for example, that you are lying on a warm, sunny beach. It is a day in midsummer and the beach is absolutely deserted. It is a beautiful spot, protected by cliffs from the wind and you have found a wonderfully secluded sun-trap between some rocks. Out at sea a yacht is anchored and you can faintly hear laughter and the tinkling of glasses. Occasionally, there is a splash as someone dives off the boat into the sea. High, high overhead you can hear seagulls calling. Just a few yards away the sea is breaking on the sandy shore. It is a wonderfully rhythmic sound, very soft and soothing.

The most insistent sensation is that of warmth. Beneath you the sand is warm. The sun is warm on your skin. Your eyes are closed and you can feel the sun on your eyelids. It is very restful to be bathed so totally in warmth. You lie there quite still and peaceful, soaking up the sun and enjoying the afternoon warmth.

Try to picture yourself from above. Look down on yourself lying there on the beach. Try to see the yellow sand. You are stretched out on a towel – dressed in just a flattering bathing costume. You look fit and strong and slim. You can tell that you no longer have any problems with your back.

I want you to see yourself looking slim and slender – just as slim as you have always dreamt of being. Imagine yourself looking the way you have always wanted to look.

You look good in your bathing costume and you know that you will look good whatever clothes you choose to wear. You see yourself roll over on your towel. You move easily and comfortably. There is no stiffness in your back or joints and clearly no pain. You can feel proud of yourself, proud of your body, proud of yourself for beating the temptations to overeat. You know that now you only ever eat because you are hungry. You never eat because you are bored, sad or unhappy. Losing your unwanted weight has made you look good and feel good, and has helped to banish your back problem for ever.

Look down and see yourself with the sort of figure you have always wanted. See yourself as a dieting success. As you look down remember the secrets of your slimming success.

Remember that you should only ever eat because you are hungry and never out of habit or boredom. Remember that every time you put food into your mouth you must ask yourself if you are really hungry. If you aren't hungry then don't eat. It is that simple.

Losing weight – and keeping your weight steady – and therefore helping your back to get stronger, really is easy. You can understand how simple it is. You eat when you are hungry. You stop when you are no longer hungry. You never eat because you are bored. You never eat because you are unhappy or miserable. You only eat when you are genuinely hungry.

Look down at yourself this one last time. Now allow yourself to go back into your body. You can feel the warmth of the sun again. You can feel the soft sand beneath you and hear the sound of the waves in the distance. You know that this is all a dream but you know now that it is an attainable dream. It is a dream that is getting closer to reality every day.

Very slowly, open your eyes. Take your time. Do it slowly and remember what you have just heard.

THE TWENTY-FIVE BEST SLIMMING TIPS

1. GIVE UP EATING MEALS. EATING FIVE OR SIX SMALL SNACKS INSTEAD OF THREE LARGE MEALS WILL HELP YOUR BODY ADJUST ITS CALORIE INTAKE TO ITS NEEDS. PEOPLE WHO 'SNACK' LOSE WEIGHT MUCH MORE SUCCESSFULLY THAN PEOPLE WHO OVER-FILL THEMSELVES WITH FOOD THREE OR FOUR TIMES A DAY.

2. STAND UP FOR YOURSELF. DON'T LET OTHER PEOPLE DECIDE WHAT YOU EAT (OR WHEN YOU EAT IT). IF YOU'RE FULL – SAY SO!

3. SET YOURSELF EASY SLIMMING TARGETS. SLIMMERS WHO TRY TO GET RID OF ALL THEIR EXCESS WEIGHT IN A MONTH WILL FAIL – AS WILL PEOPLE WHO TRY TO LOSE TOO MUCH WEIGHT. DECIDE WHAT YOUR IDEAL WEIGHT SHOULD BE AND THEN AIM AT LOSING TWO POUNDS A WEEK.

4. ONLY EVER EAT WHEN YOU ARE HUNGRY, AND STOP WHEN YOU ARE FULL. EVERY TIME YOU ARE ABOUT TO PUT FOOD INTO YOUR MOUTH ASK YOURSELF WHETHER OR NOT YOU REALLY NEED IT.

5. DON'T EAT IN THE EVENING. IF YOU EAT WHEN YOU'RE SITTING DOWN – OR ABOUT TO GO TO BED – YOUR BODY WILL STORE THE UNWANTED CALORIES AS FAT. YOU SHOULD CONSUME MOST OF YOUR FOOD EARLY IN THE DAY – SO THAT YOUR BODY CAN BURN UP THE CALORIES.

6. START A COMPOST HEAP. NEVER BE AFRAID TO THROW FOOD AWAY IF YOU DON'T WANT IT. MOST PEOPLE WHO HAVE A WEIGHT PROBLEM HATE SEEING FOOD WASTED AND WILL FINISH UP THE SCRAPS OFF OTHER PEOPLES' PLATES RATHER THAN DUMP UNWANTED FOOD INTO THE BIN.

7. TAKE REGULAR EXERCISE. IT WILL HELP TONE UP YOUR MUSCLES AND BURN UP A FEW EXTRA CALORIES. SWIMMING AND WALKING ARE BOTH EXCELLENT FORMS OF EXERCISE AND STRESS FREE.

8. DON'T WORRY ABOUT WEIGHING FOOD OR COUNTING CALORIES. ALLOW YOUR BODY TO HELP YOU DIET SUCCESSFULLY BY DECIDING WHEN – AND HOW MUCH – YOU NEED TO EAT.

9. IF YOU FEEL HUNGRY AND FIND YOURSELF REACHING FOR FOOD WAIT FIVE MINUTES. THEN – IF YOU *STILL* FEEL HUNGRY – YOU CAN EAT.

10. WHEN YOU SIT DOWN TO A MEAL DO NOT IMMEDIATELY START SHOVELLING FOOD INTO YOUR MOUTH. SIT FOR A MOMENT OR TWO AND RELAX. TRY TO GET RID OF ACCUMULATED TENSIONS. THEN EAT SLOWLY AND CONCENTRATE ON

WHAT YOU ARE DOING. THIS WAY YOU WILL BE FAR MORE LIKELY TO HEAR YOUR BODY 'TALKING' TO YOU.

11. STOP BETWEEN COURSES AND REST. IF YOU'VE HAD ENOUGH TO EAT GET UP AND LEAVE THE TABLE. NEVER STAY SITTING AT THE TABLE AFTER YOU'VE FINISHED EATING OR ELSE THERE IS A RISK THAT YOU WILL NIBBLE AT WHATEVER IS LEFT.

12. USE SWEETENERS INSTEAD OF SUGAR. BY MAKING THIS SIMPLE SUBSTITUTION MOST PEOPLE CAN LOSE OVER 14 POUNDS A YEAR.

13. NEVER REWARD YOURSELF WITH FOOD. IF YOU ARE PLEASED OR PROUD OR YOU WANT TO CELEBRATE, DO SO WITH A BUNCH OF FLOWERS, A NEW TAPE OR A BOOK OR MAGAZINE. FOOD IS FOR EATING.

14. DON'T SPEND TOO MUCH TIME *LOOKING* AT MOUTH-WATERING FOOD. THERE IS EVIDENCE NOW TO SHOW THAT YOU CAN GET FAT JUST BY LOOKING. WHEN YOU SEE, SMELL OR THINK OF FOOD YOUR BODY STARTS TO PREPARE ITS DIGESTIVE PROCESSES. SALIVA IS RELEASED IN YOUR MOUTH AND YOUR STOMACH PRODUCES JUICES TO HELP DIGEST THE COMING FOOD. THE PANCREAS IS STIMULATED AND INSULIN IS PRODUCED. THE INSULIN THEN STARTS TO CONVERT THE GLUCOSE IN YOUR BLOODSTREAM INTO FAT AS YOUR BODY CLEARS THE WAY FOR THE FOOD IT THINKS IS ON THE WAY. HOWEVER, AS THE AMOUNT OF SUGAR IN YOUR BLOOD FALLS SO YOU WILL BEGIN TO FEEL GENUINELY HUNGRY, AND YOU WILL NEED TO EAT. YOUR BODY WILL HAVE BEEN TRICKED BY ITS OWN SENSES.

15. DON'T WEIGH YOURSELF EVERY DAY. ONCE A WEEK IS ENOUGH. YOUR WEIGHT WILL VARY DAILY FOR ALL SORTS OF REASONS AND YOU ARE LIKELY TO BECOME OBSESSED OR DEPRESSED IF YOU WEIGH YOURSELF TOO OFTEN.

16. IF YOU FIND SLIMMING ALONE TOO DIFFICULT, CONSIDER JOINING A SLIMMING CLUB. THERE ARE HUNDREDS OF THEM AROUND. LOOK IN THE LOCAL TELEPHONE BOOK OR ASK YOUR DOCTOR. MANY PEOPLE GET SUPPORT AND ENCOURAGEMENT FROM SLIMMING WITH OTHERS.

17. SPEND A LITTLE TIME WORKING OUT HOW YOU ACQUIRED YOUR BAD EATING HABITS. WHAT BAD EATING HABITS DID YOU LEARN AS A CHILD? AWARENESS OF YOUR BAD EATING HABITS WILL MAKE THEM EASIER TO CONQUER.

18. EAT MOST OF YOUR MEALS SITTING AT THE TABLE. NEVER EAT IN FRONT OF THE TV SET. YOU NEED TO CONCENTRATE ON WHAT YOU ARE DOING IF YOU ARE GOING TO USE THE POWER OF YOUR MIND TO HELP YOU SLIM

SUCCESSFULLY. DO NOT CARRY FOOD AROUND YOUR HOME – EAT ONLY IN THE KITCHEN OR DINING ROOM.

19. DO NOT FOLLOW ANY 'MAGICAL' OR 'WONDER' DIETS YOU SEE ADVERTISED THAT PROMISE YOU INSTANT SLENDERNESS, AND DON'T WASTE YOUR MONEY ON SLIMMING PILLS OR SUPPLEMENTS.

20. IF YOU HAVE TO ATTEND A BIG DINNER OR CELEBRATION MEAL AND YOU ARE WORRIED THAT IT WILL RUIN YOUR DIET HAVE A SNACK HALF AN HOUR BEFOREHAND. IT WILL SPOIL YOUR APPETITE AND ENSURE THAT YOU FEEL FULL LONG BEFORE YOU DO YOUR DIET TOO MUCH DAMAGE.

21. DO NOT BE ATTEMPTED TO NIBBLE WHILE YOU ARE COOKING. MANY COOKS PERSUADE THEMSELVES THAT THEY ARE TESTING FOOD AS THEY COOK, BUT BY THE TIME THE MEAL IS READY THEY WILL HAVE EATEN FAR MORE THAN A 'SAMPLE'. THEY THEN SIT DOWN, HAVE A SMALL MEAL AND CONVINCE THEMSELVES THAT THEY HAVE EATEN HARDLY ANYTHING. THIS SORT OF NIBBLING HAS NOTHING AT ALL TO DO WITH HUNGER.

22. MANY PRESCRIBED PILLS CAN PRODUCE AN UNWANTED WEIGHT GAIN. DRUGS SUCH AS STEROIDS CAN DO THIS. IF YOU ARE REGULARLY TAKING ANY PRESCRIBED PILL AND YOU SUSPECT THAT IT COULD BE DAMAGING YOUR ATTEMPTS AT DIETING TALK TO YOUR DOCTOR. THERE MAY BE AN ALTERNATIVE THAT HE CAN PRESCRIBE.

23. START BUYING CLOTHES THAT YOU WILL ONLY BE ABLE TO WEAR WHEN YOU HAVE LOST WEIGHT. KEEP LOOKING AT THE CLOTHES AND IMAGINE YOURSELF WEARING THEM. THINK ABOUT THE MONEY YOU WILL HAVE WASTED IF YOU ARE NOT ABLE TO WEAR THEM BEFORE THEY GO OUT OF FASHION. YOU WILL FIND THIS A TREMENDOUS INCENTIVE TO LOSE WEIGHT.

24. ALWAYS BE POSITIVE WHEN YOU ARE TALKING ABOUT YOUR EATING HABITS. IF SOMEONE SAYS TO YOU 'ARE YOU TRYING TO DIET?' SAY 'NO I HAVE DECIDED TO CHANGE MY EATING HABITS AND LOSE SOME WEIGHT.' THE WORD 'TRY' SUGGESTS THE POSSIBILITY OF FAILURE. YOU ARE NOT GOING TO FAIL TO LOSE WEIGHT.

25. MAKE YOUR RIGHT HAND INTO A FIST. THIS IS THE APPROXIMATE SIZE OF YOUR STOMACH. EVEN IF YOU WERE STARVING THE AMOUNT OF FOOD YOU WOULD NEED TO SATISFY YOUR HUNGER WOULD ONLY FILL A CONTAINER THE SIZE OF YOUR FIST. REMEMBER THAT THE NEXT TIME YOU ARE TEMPTED TO EAT YOUR WAY THROUGH A HUGE PLATE FULL OF FOOD AND INSTEAD EAT JUST ENOUGH TO FILL THAT IMAGINARY CONTAINER.

HOW MUCH SHOULD YOU WEIGH?

INSTRUCTIONS
1. WEIGH YOURSELF WITH AS FEW CLOTHES AS POSSIBLE – AND NO SHOES.
2. MEASURE YOUR HEIGHT IN BARE OR STOCKINGED FEET.
3. YOU ARE OVERWEIGHT IF YOUR WEIGHT FALLS ABOVE YOUR IDEAL WEIGHT BAND AND YOUR BACK WILL BENEFIT IF YOU LOSE WEIGHT.

HEIGHT/WEIGHT CHART

HEIGHT (FEET & INCHES)
IDEAL WEIGHT BAND (STONES & POUNDS)

FOR WOMEN			FOR MEN		
4.10	7.5 –	8.5	5.0	8.5 –	9.5
4.11	7.7 –	8.7	5.1	8.6 –	9.6
5.0	7.9 –	8.9	5.2	8.7 –	9.7
5.1	7.11 –	8.11	5.3	8.8 –	9.8
5.2	8.1 –	9.1	5.4	8.11 –	9.11
5.3	8.4 –	9.4	5.5	9.2 –	10.2
5.4	8.6 –	9.6	5.6	9.6 –	10.6
5.5	8.10 –	9.10	5.7	9.10 –	10.10
5.6	9.0 –	10.0	5.8	10.0 –	11.0
5.7	9.3 –	10.3	5.9	10.4 –	11.4
5.8	9.7 –	10.7	5.10	10.8 –	11.8
5.9	9.10 –	10.10	5.11	10.12 –	11.12
5.10	10.0 –	11.0	6.0	11.2 –	12.2
5.11	10.3 –	11.3	6.1	11.6 –	12.6
6.0	10.7 –	11.7	6.2	11.10 –	12.10
6.1	10.9 –	11.9	6.3	12.0 –	13.0
6.2	10.12 –	11.12	6.4	12.4 –	13.4
6.3	11.2 –	12.2	6.5	12.8 –	13.8
6.4	11.5 –	12.5	6.6	13.0 –	14.0
6.5	11.8 –	12.8			
6.6	12.0 –	13.0			

NOTE: IDEAL WEIGHTS VARY WITH AGE AND VARIOUS OTHER FACTORS. BUT IF YOU WEIGH MORE THAN 14 POUNDS ABOVE THE MAXIMUM IN YOUR IDEAL WEIGHT BAND THEN YOUR WEIGHT WILL ALMOST CERTAINLY BE HAVING AN ADVERSE EFFECT ON YOUR BACK.

CHAPTER FOUR

Exercises For Your Back

THE TRUTH ABOUT EXERCISE

Do you take enough exercise?

The chances are high that you don't, and the chances are high that one of the reasons why you suffer so much from back trouble is because you do not exercise enough.

By itself exercise might not stop you getting back pains, but it certainly could help strengthen your general level of fitness, increase your resistance to muscular stresses and strains, and reduce your susceptibility to backache.

You could help reduce the amount of backache from which you suffer simply by exercising your back muscles, but that would be rather short-sighted.

"Are you one of those people who is forever planning to start a fitness programme but just always seems to be too busy, or finds it more convenient to start the next week?"

The fact is that if you have not been doing enough exercise then you also need to start a good, general exercise programme to improve your general strength and health, as well as performing exercises to improve the strength and health of your back.

In this chapter I've provided the information to help you do both!

Are you one of those people who is forever planning to start a fitness programme but just always seems to be too busy, or finds it more convenient to start the next week but never does? But beware. If your enthusiasm gets the better of you and you suddenly throw yourself into a hectic exercise programme you could do yourself more harm than good.

However, unless you take regular exercise you may jeopardize your general health and in addition to getting backache you will be more prone to disorders as varied as arthritis, osteoporosis, heart disease and depression.

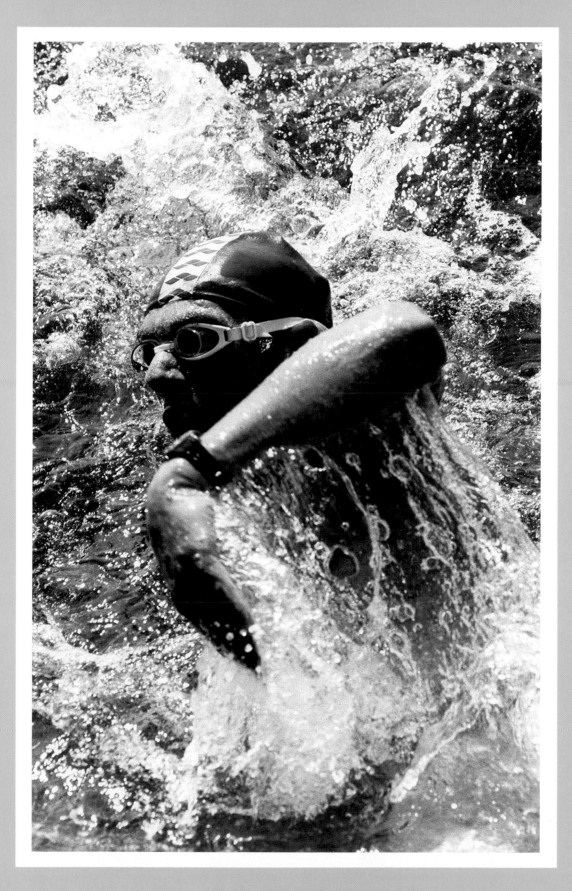

THE BENEFITS OF EXERCISE

EXERCISE IS VITALLY IMPORTANT FOR A NUMBER OF REASONS. HERE ARE JUST SOME OF THE WAYS IN WHICH A WELL THOUGHT-OUT GENERAL EXERCISE PROGRAMME CAN HELP IMPROVE YOUR HEALTH:

1. STRESS AND TENSION ARE POTENTIALLY VERY HARMFUL. EXERCISE IS WITHOUT DOUBT ONE OF THE BEST WAYS OF FIGHTING THE DAMAGING EFFECTS OF ANXIETY AND WORRY.

2. REGULAR EXERCISE WILL HELP TO KEEP YOUR JOINTS SUPPLE AND THUS DELAY THE ONSET OF SUCH DISEASES AS ARTHRITIS.

3. REGULAR EXERCISE WILL HELP TO GET RID OF TENSION IN THE MUSCLES AROUND YOUR HEAD AND WILL PREVENT TENSION HEADACHES.

4. A GOOD EXERCISE PROGRAMME WILL HELP TO ENSURE THAT THE BLOOD DOES NOT STAGNATE IN YOUR VEINS. EXERCISE CAN HELP TO IMPROVE YOUR CIRCULATION AND PREVENT COLD FEET, COLD HANDS AND VARICOSE VEINS.

5. THE PHYSICAL TIREDNESS WHICH RESULTS FROM EXERCISE MAKES FOR A BETTER NIGHT'S SLEEP. THIS MEANS THAT REGULAR EXERCISE COULD TAKE AWAY THE NEED FOR SLEEPING PILLS.

6. SINCE YOUR WEIGHT IS A CONSEQUENCE OF THE AMOUNT OF FOOD YOU EAT, AND THE AMOUNT OF EXERCISE YOU DO, A REGULAR EXERCISE PROGRAMME WILL HELP YOU BURN FOOD UP FASTER WITH THE RESULT THAT YOU WILL GET SLIMMER. REGULAR EXERCISE WILL ALSO HELP TO TONE UP YOUR MUSCLES, MAKING YOU LOOK SLIMMER.

7. IF YOU DO NOT DO ANY EXERCISE YOUR HEART WILL BECOME FLABBY AND WEAK. A WELL-ORGANIZED EXERCISE PROGRAMME WILL STRENGTHEN YOUR HEART AND REDUCE YOUR CHANCES OF SUFFERING FROM HEART DISEASE.

8. SINCE A SEDENTARY LIFESTYLE, SITTING OR EVEN STANDING IN ONE POSITION FOR A LONG TIME CAN LEAD TO BACKACHE, A GOOD EXERCISE PROGRAMME (PARTICULARLY ONE WHICH HELPS TO KEEP YOUR BACK SUPPLE AND STRONG) WILL HELP REDUCE YOUR CHANCES OF SUFFERING FROM BACK TROUBLE.

9. DIGESTIVE DISORDERS SUCH AS THE IRRITABLE BOWEL SYNDROME CAN BE HELPED OR ALLEVIATED BY WELL-ORGANIZED, REGULAR EXERCISE.

10. A REGULAR EXERCISE PROGRAMME WILL HELP YOU TO STAY CHEERFUL AND FIGHT BOUTS OF SADNESS OR MILD DEPRESSION.

We live in a technological age which provides little opportunity for physical exertion. We travel in cars, buses and trains, and we use all sorts of labour-saving devices to help us cut down the workload in the house and garden. Very few of us make any effort to exercise regularly. We may play the occasional game of football, take the occasional Sunday afternoon stroll or enjoy swimming on a holiday in the sun, but that really isn't good enough. Our bodies have evolved more slowly than the world around us and are still designed for action. Bodies needs exercise, and just as important they need regular exercise. Many of the diseases that are common today are partly caused by the fact that most of us simply do not exercise enough.

However, before getting fired with enthusiasm and rushing off to the nearest aerobics class or off for a cross-country run there are some important points which need to be considered. How much exercise is good for you and how often should you exercise? Do you have any illnesses or ailments which may be exacerbated rather than helped by exercise? Remember the most important rule for exercise: it should never hurt. Pain is your body's way of saying 'Stop'. If you ignore a pain and attempt to blunder bravely through the pain barrier, you will almost certainly injure yourself.

It is very important to check with your doctor if you are in any doubt about your fitness to undertake an exercise programme. Be sensible. Start exercising gently. A short session two or three times a week is fine to start with. You may find it more encouraging to exercise with other people so it is probably best to try to find a gym with a good coach, a well-run aerobics class or a sports club that you can join. A good coach may assess your fitness, suggest a programme for you to follow and show you how to take your pulse before and after every exercise session. Within a few weeks you should notice that your pulse will go back to its normal rate more and more quickly after exercising and that your normal rate will get lower as you get fitter. See the chart on page 61 which shows the range within which you should keep your pulse when you exercise.

It is important to set aside time for a properly organized exercise programme, otherwise you will always be trying to find excuses to avoid exercising. Regular exercise should become part of your weekly routine. Try to give it priority over other less vital tasks.

It need not be much – three sessions a week of an hour each will be quite sufficient, and you may want to start with less and build up to three hours a week. If you are really pushed for time you can squeeze a useful exercise programme into just three 20-minute sessions.

You don't need a lot of money to take up exercise but you do need to buy the right shoes and comfortable clothes – the best you can afford. Remember the gym is not the catwalk, but you do need shoes that are comfortable and give good support, and since you will be sweating a lot when you start exercising properly you will need clothes that can be washed and dried often, quickly and easily.

WARNING

1. DO NOT START AN EXERCISE PROGRAMME UNTIL YOU HAVE CHECKED WITH YOUR DOCTOR THAT IT IS SUITABLE FOR YOU. MAKE SURE THAT YOU TELL HIM ABOUT ANY TREATMENT YOU ARE ALREADY RECEIVING AND ABOUT ANY SYMPTOMS FROM WHICH YOU SUFFER.

2. YOU MUST STOP EXERCISING IF YOU FEEL FAINT, DIZZY, BREATHLESS OR NAUSEATED, OR IF YOU NOTICE ANY PAIN OR FEEL UNWELL IN ANY WAY. GET EXPERT HELP IMMEDIATELY AND DO NOT START EXERCISING AGAIN UNTIL YOU HAVE BEEN GIVEN THE 'ALL CLEAR' BY YOUR DOCTOR.

EXERCISES TO STRENGTHEN YOUR BACK

The exercises on the following pages will help improve the strength of your back, but before trying any of them do check first with your doctor. You should try to repeat each individual exercise five to ten times – but stop at once if you get the slightest pain or discomfort. You should not do any of these exercises if you are already in pain, receiving treatment of any kind or if you have had or are awaiting surgery. Remember: you must always check with your doctor before doing any exercises or before starting any exercise programme.

EXERCISES TO IMPROVE THE STRENGTH OF YOUR LOWER BACK MUSCLES

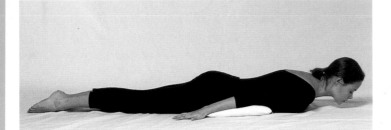

1. *PUT A FAIRLY FIRM PILLOW OR CUSHION ON THE FLOOR AND LIE FACE DOWN WITH YOUR TUMMY ON THE PILLOW. THEN LIFT YOUR HEAD AND SHOULDERS TO THE HORIZONTAL. DO THIS MOVEMENT WITHOUT ARCHING YOUR BACK.*

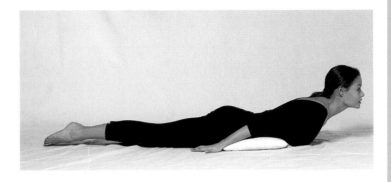

2. *PUT A THIN PILLOW OR FOLDED TOWEL ON THE EDGE OF A FIRM, STRONG, STABLE TABLE. NOW LIE FORWARD ON THE TABLE SO THAT YOUR HIPS ARE RESTING ON THE PILLOW OR TOWEL. HOLD ONTO THE EDGES OF THE TABLE WITH YOUR HANDS AND LIFT YOUR LEGS UP TO THE HORIZONTAL POSITION.*

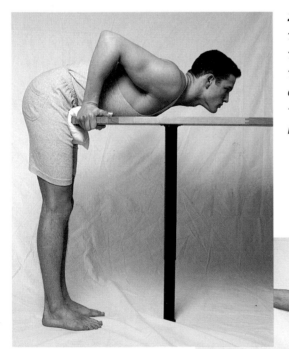

EXERCISES TO STRENGTHEN YOUR ABDOMINAL MUSCLES

1. *LIE ON YOUR BACK ON THE FLOOR WITH YOUR FEET FLAT ON THE FLOOR AND YOUR KNEES BENT. REST YOUR RIGHT HAND ON YOUR ABDOMEN. NOW TAKE A DEEP BREATH IN AND AS YOU BREATHE OUT GENTLY PULL IN YOUR ABDOMINAL MUSCLES. ONCE YOU KNOW WHAT IT FEELS LIKE TO CONTRACT YOUR ABDOMINAL MUSCLES YOU CAN REPEAT THIS VERY SIMPLE EXERCISE REGULARLY THROUGHOUT THE DAY. THE STRONGER YOU CAN MAKE YOUR ABDOMINAL MUSCLES THE BETTER WILL BE THE PROTECTION YOUR BACK GETS.*

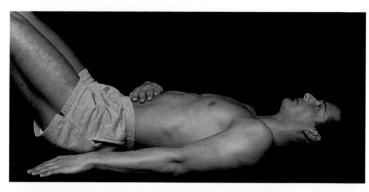

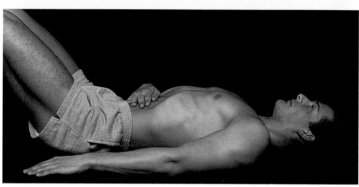

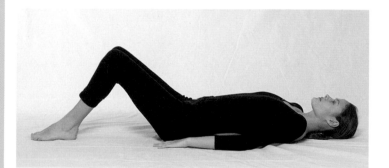

2. *LIE ON YOUR BACK ON THE FLOOR WITH YOUR FEET FLAT ON THE FLOOR AND YOUR KNEES BENT. NOW LIFT YOUR HEAD AND SHOULDERS, STRETCH OUT YOUR ARMS AND REACH FORWARDS AND TRY TO TOUCH YOUR KNEES.*

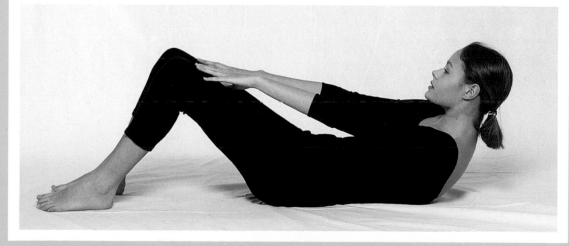

EXERCISES TO STRENGTHEN YOUR ABDOMINAL MUSCLES (CONTINUED)

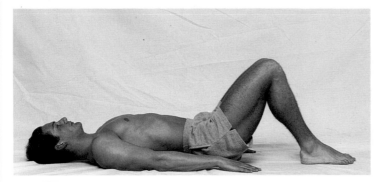

4. *LIE ON YOUR BACK ON THE FLOOR WITH YOUR FEET FLAT ON THE FLOOR AND YOUR KNEES BENT. PUT YOUR ARMS DOWN BY YOUR SIDES WITH YOUR PALMS FLAT ON THE FLOOR.*

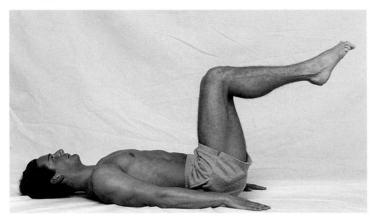

NOW PULL BOTH YOUR KNEES UP TOWARDS YOUR CHEST.

THEN STRAIGHTEN YOUR LEGS SO THAT YOUR FEET ARE POINTING TO THE CEILING. THEN BRING YOUR KNEES BACK DOWN AGAIN AND PUT YOUR FEET BACK ON THE FLOOR.

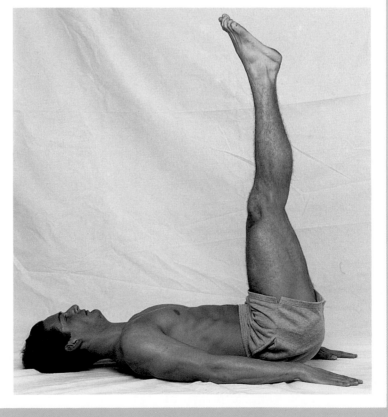

5. LIE ON YOUR BACK ON THE FLOOR WITH YOUR FEET FLAT ON THE FLOOR AND YOUR KNEES BENT. PUT YOUR ARMS DOWN BY YOUR SIDES WITH YOUR PALMS FLAT ON THE FLOOR.

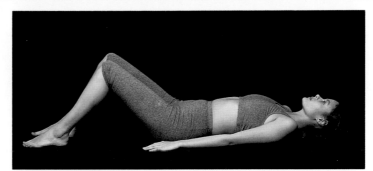

NOW PULL YOUR KNEES RIGHT UP TO YOUR CHEST.

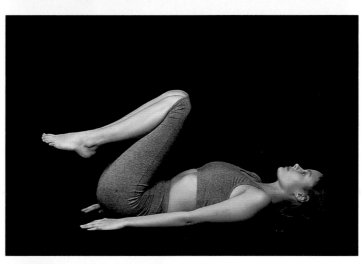

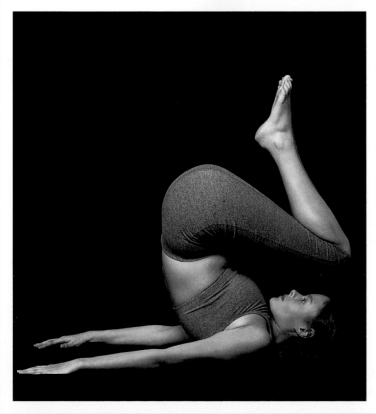

FINALLY TRY TO LIFT YOUR BOTTOM RIGHT OFF THE FLOOR. TRY TO GET YOUR KNEES AS CLOSE TO YOUR HEAD AS YOU CAN, BUT REMEMBER TO STOP IMMEDIATELY IF YOU FEEL ANY DISCOMFORT OR PAIN.

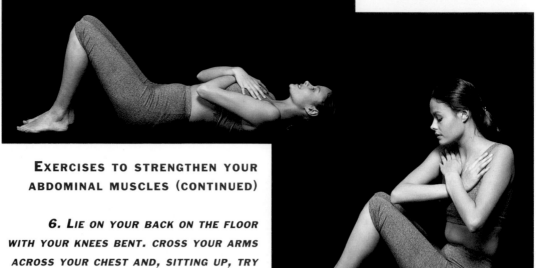

EXERCISES TO STRENGTHEN YOUR ABDOMINAL MUSCLES (CONTINUED)

6. LIE ON YOUR BACK ON THE FLOOR WITH YOUR KNEES BENT. CROSS YOUR ARMS ACROSS YOUR CHEST AND, SITTING UP, TRY TO TOUCH YOUR RIGHT KNEE WITH YOUR LEFT ELBOW AND YOUR LEFT KNEE WITH YOUR RIGHT ELBOW.

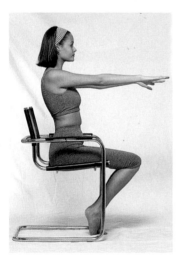

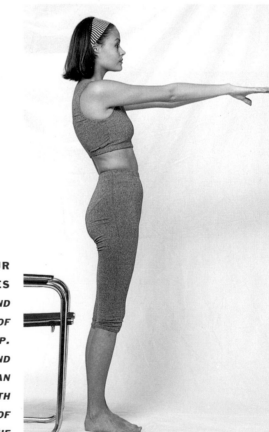

EXERCISES TO STRENGTHEN YOUR LEG MUSCLES

1. SIT ON AN ORDINARY DINING CHAIR AND HOLD YOUR ARMS STRAIGHT OUT IN FRONT OF YOU. THEN STAND UP. SIT DOWN. STAND UP. SIT DOWN. DO THIS TEN TIMES. IF YOU FIND IT TOO EASY TO STAND UP FROM AN ORDINARY CHAIR TRY STANDING UP WITH YOUR ARMS HELD STRAIGHT OUT IN FRONT OF YOU FROM SITTING ON A LOW STOOL OR THE BOTTOM STEP OF A STAIRCASE.

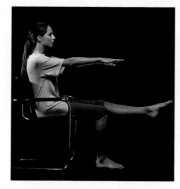

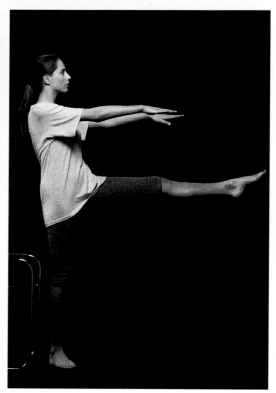

2. S*IT ON AN ORDINARY DINING CHAIR AND HOLD YOUR ARMS STRAIGHT OUT IN FRONT OF YOU. L*IFT YOUR LEFT LEG UNTIL IT IS HORIZONTAL TO THE FLOOR. N*OW STAND UP, USING ONLY YOUR RIGHT LEG. A*LTERNATE RIGHT AND LEFT LEGS. I*F YOU FIND THIS TOO EASY YOU CAN TRY IT FROM A SITTING POSITION ON A LOW STOOL OR THE BOTTOM STEP OF A STAIRCASE. D*O NOT TRY THIS EXERCISE IF YOU THINK YOU ARE LIKELY TO OVERBALANCE.*

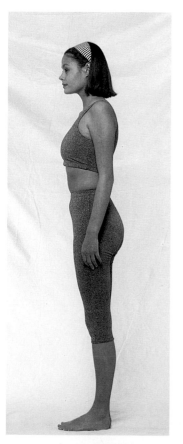

3. S*TAND WITH YOUR FEET SLIGHTLY APART. K*EEPING YOUR SPINE AS STRAIGHT AS YOU CAN AND YOUR KNEES TOGETHER SLOWLY BEND AT THE KNEES UNTIL YOU ARE SQUATTING. S*LOWLY STAND UP. H*OLD ON TO A PIECE OF STABLE FURNITURE IF YOU NEED TO.*

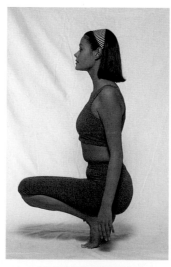

Exercises to stretch your back and make it more mobile

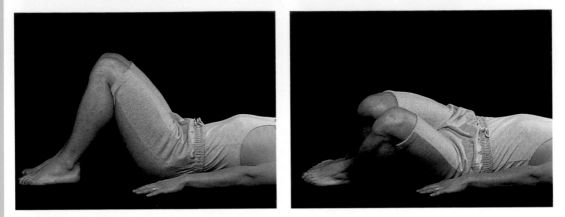

1. Lie flat on your back on the floor with your knees bent and your feet flat on the floor. Then lower both knees, first to the right and then to the left.

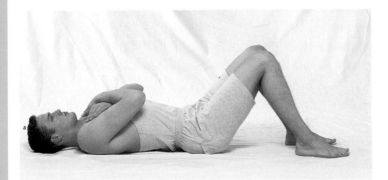

2. Lie flat on your back on the floor with your knees bent and your feet flat on the floor. Then lift your bottom as high as you can. Hold it there for two or three seconds then lower it down again.

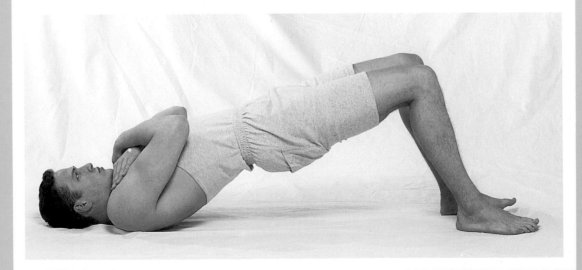

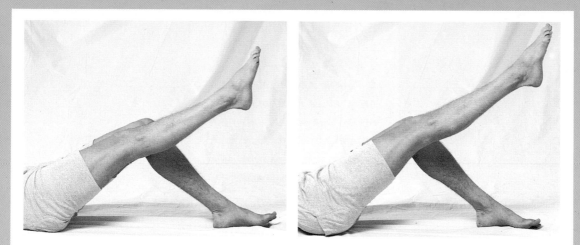

3. LIE FLAT ON YOUR BACK ON THE FLOOR WITH YOUR KNEES BENT AND YOUR FEET FLAT ON THE FLOOR. THEN STRAIGHTEN YOUR RIGHT LEG AND ALTERNATELY MAKE IT AS LONG AND AS SHORT AS YOU CAN. DO THE SAME WITH YOUR LEFT LEG.

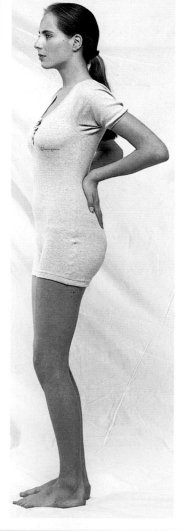

4. STAND UP STRAIGHT WITH YOUR FEET ABOUT SHOULDER-WIDTH APART AND POINTING FORWARDS. PUT YOUR HANDS IN THE SMALL OF YOUR BACK AND BREATHE IN DEEPLY. BREATHE OUT SLOWLY AND BEND BACKWARDS, SUPPORTING YOUR BACK WITH YOUR HANDS.

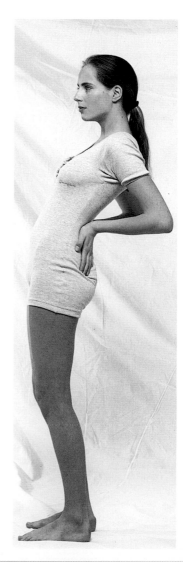

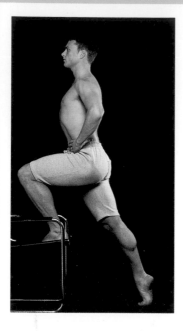

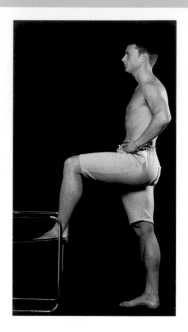

EXERCISES TO STRETCH YOUR BACK (CONTINUED)

5. STAND ABOUT ONE FOOT AWAY FROM AN ORDINARY DINING CHAIR. LIFT ONE FOOT UP AND PUT IT FLAT ON THE CHAIR. LEAN FORWARDS AND YOU SHOULD FEEL YOUR OTHER LEG STRETCHING. THEN CHANGE LEGS.

6. STAND ABOUT TWO OR THREE FEET AWAY FROM AN ORDINARY DINING CHAIR. LIFT YOUR RIGHT FOOT AND PUT YOUR HEEL ON THE CHAIR. KEEP YOUR OUTSTRETCHED LEG STRAIGHT AND BEND THE LEG YOU ARE STANDING ON. THEN CHANGE LEGS.

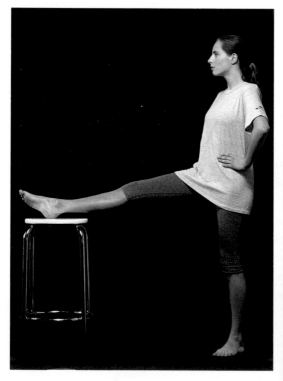

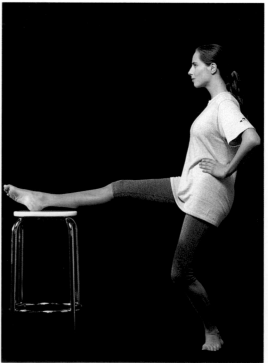

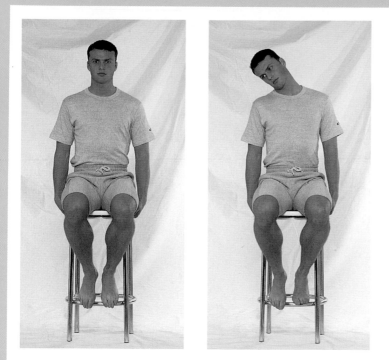

7. SIT DOWN ON AN ORDINARY DINING CHAIR, HOLDING THE UNDERSIDE OF THE CHAIR WITH YOUR HANDS. KEEP YOUR RIGHT ARM STRAIGHT AND YOUR SHOULDER STABLE AND LEAN YOUR HEAD AS FAR TO THE LEFT AS YOU CAN. HOLD THE STRETCH FOR AS LONG AS POSSIBLE AND THEN LEAN YOUR HEAD AS FAR TO THE RIGHT AS YOU CAN.

QUICK AND SIMPLE EXERCISES TO HELP STRENGTHEN YOUR BACK

NOTE: ONCE AGAIN DO NOT TRY THESE EXERCISES IF YOU ARE SUFFERING FROM BACKACHE OR ANY OTHER PROBLEM. TALK TO YOUR DOCTOR BEFORE TRYING ANY EXERCISE PROGRAMME.

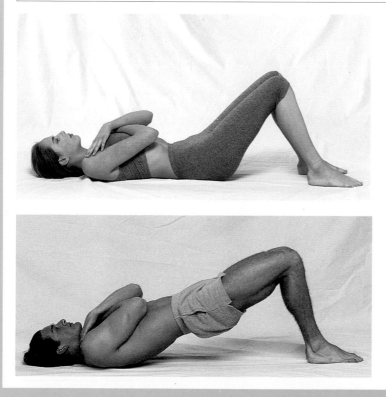

FOR THE FOLLOWING FIVE EXERCISES LIE FLAT ON YOUR BACK WITH YOUR KNEES BENT, YOUR FEET FLAT ON THE FLOOR AND YOUR ARMS FOLDED ACROSS YOUR CHEST. THEN:

1. PULL IN YOUR TUMMY MUSCLES AS FAR AS THEY WILL GO. DO THIS FIVE TIMES.

2. LIFT YOUR BOTTOM OFF THE FLOOR – AS HIGH AS YOU CAN. DO THIS FIVE TIMES.

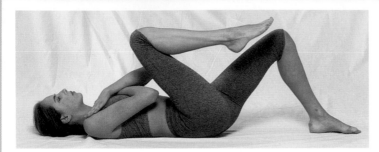

3. BRING YOUR RIGHT KNEE AS CLOSE TO YOUR CHEST AS YOU CAN. DO THIS FIVE TIMES.

4. DO EXERCISE 3 WITH YOUR LEFT KNEE. REPEAT FIVE TIMES.

5. TRY TO SIT UP AND TOUCH YOUR KNEES. REPEAT FIVE TIMES. NOW STAND UP:

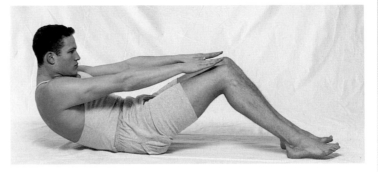

REMEMBER: STOP IF ANY EXERCISE IS PAINFUL. NEVER STRAIN. WITH YOUR DOCTOR'S PERMISSION YOU SHOULD REPEAT THIS SIMPLE EXERCISE PROGRAMME TWICE A DAY – EVERY DAY.

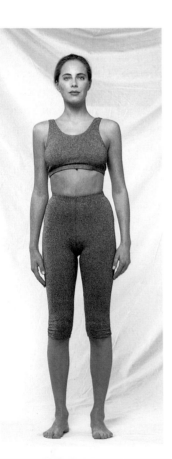

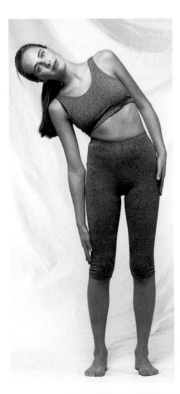

PUT YOUR FEET APART. BEND YOUR BODY TO YOUR RIGHT AND TRY TO TOUCH YOUR RIGHT KNEE WITH YOUR RIGHT HAND. THEN BEND YOUR BODY THE OTHER WAY AND TRY TO TOUCH YOUR LEFT KNEE WITH YOUR LEFT HAND. REPEAT FIVE TIMES.

EXERCISES TO BEWARE OF!

Some stretching and muscle strengthening exercises are particularly likely to cause back problems. You should always take great care to make sure that you never do any exercises which cause any pain at all, and if you have a back problem or a history of back trouble you should talk to your doctor before beginning to exercise (however gentle or safe it may seem to be). Here are some specific exercises that are among those which are especially likely to cause problems.

TOUCHING YOUR TOES

This common exercise can put a strain on your back. It is even more likely to damage your spine if you put a twist into the exercise by attempting to touch your right foot with your left hand and then your left foot with your right hand.

BENDING FORWARDS

Exercises which involve a forwards movement are designed to strengthen your abdominal muscles. If you have a prolapsed disc, however, this exercise can damage your spinal cord.

SPINE-STRETCHING EXERCISES

Too much stretching can damage and weaken the joints which connect the separate vertebrae.

BENDING SIDEWAYS

Although exercise can be helpful it needs to be done carefully, slowly and over a short range if you are to avoid excessive rotation of the vertebrae.

TWISTING EXERCISES

The idea is that by twisting you can mobilize stiff joints. But if you have joints in your spine that are completely immobile the result will be to overstrain your other spinal joints.

RAISING BOTH LEGS

This exercise is often recommended as good for strengthening the muscles of the abdomen. But it does put quite a strain on the lower back. Do not attempt it if it is painful or if you have a weak or injured back.

THE WRONG SORT OF EXERCISE CAN DAMAGE YOUR BACK

Although exercise is essential for a healthy back it can cause problems. Your back consists of many separate joints and all of those joints can be put under a tremendous amount of strain by any repetitive exercise. As a result backache is a common problem among sportsmen and athletes who do not take care. Warming up beforehand, resting or even stopping when you feel tired and cooling down gently after an exercise programme are all very important.

Running is one of the sports most commonly associated with back injury. Running tends to tighten the lower muscles of the back causing low back pain and increasing the risk of conditions such as ruptured disc or spondylolysis, and runners who exercise for too long on hard surfaces are particularly likely to suffer from backache. Every one hour's running means that the back gets 10,000 vibrations it doesn't want. Running on cambered roads means that the strains on the back are particularly bad because one leg is always running lower than the other.

Running is not, of course, the only sport that can cause back problems. Virtually any sport, whether energetic or not, can cause trouble. Over-enthusiastic swinging of a golf club, for example, can cause nasty strains that may take a long time to heal.

The most severe and potentially serious back injuries tend to occur in contact sports such as rugby and football or martial arts where a sudden jolt can fracture a vertebrae, damage the spinal cord and produce permanent paralysis.

Damage to the cervical spine is most common in combat sports. The current enthusiasm for karate and aikido has seen a dramatic increase in the number of such injuries. Diving, particularly into a shallow pool, can also result in serious neck injuries.

There is no doubt that taking part in sport regularly can reduce your chances of suffering from stress and heart disease, will almost certainly help to control your weight, and will improve your muscle strength and joint flexibility. But sport of almost any kind can be dangerous, and if you are susceptible to back trouble you must be careful about the type of sport you choose.

A TYPICAL CASE HISTORY

Roger P works in a bank where he has an important post, which means that he has to spend eight or ten hours a day sitting at a desk. For much of the past ten years Roger has suffered from persistent back pains.

Despite numerous X-rays and hospital investigations doctors have failed to find anything seriously wrong with his back. They could find no bone or joint abnormality and every test they did was negative.

Up until the time when I first saw him, Roger was regularly taking pain killers. Sadly, the pain killers caused problems of their own. Taking too many aspirin and codeine compounds had, over the years, led to Roger continually suffering the discomfort of both indigestion and constipation.

Roger had tried both acupuncture and homoeopathy in order to get relief from his persistent backache but although his pains were helped a little, they never went away completely. His backache was so persistent and so severe that he had to give up playing golf (which he loved) and his wife had to take over the running of their garden.

When I examined him it was clear that a good many of Roger's problems were caused by the fact that he spent most of his time sitting down and very little time exercising his muscles.

The muscles of the back play a vital part in protecting the whole structure, and Roger's muscles simply weren't strong enough to do their job properly. He was only in his early forties but he was less fit than many men in their fifties or sixties.

These problems were undoubtedly made considerably worse by the fact that Roger was noticeably and unhealthily overweight.

Using the dietary advice on pages 32 to 43, the back muscle strengthening exercises on pages 47 to 59, and the general exercise programme outlined below, Roger made a real effort both to lose his unhealthy weight and to improve his bone and muscle strength and his general fitness.

Within three months he had lost over 14 pounds (6.35 kilos) in weight and he had greatly improved his general level of fitness, his muscle strength and his flexibility. One day Roger came into my surgery with a smile on his face to tell me that he had not suffered any back pain at all for a whole week. It was the first time in years that he had gone for seven days without suffering from backache. He had not needed to take a single pain killer! He was, needless to say, delighted.

GENERAL EXERCISE PROGRAMME

The general exercise programme which appears on the following pages is suitable for use by people who have had back trouble, who have recovered and who now want to strengthen and improve their backs and their general fitness. It is important that you realize that this programme is not suitable if you are suffering from back trouble at the moment but it will help you if you are looking for a simple, relatively undemanding, easy to understand exercise programme that will improve your muscle strength, help to increase your general flexibility and improve your general fitness level.

Designed to improve your general health and fitness, this exercise programme consists of three parts:

1. Aerobics. This part is designed to improve your general level of fitness.

2. Weight training. This will improve the strength and therefore the stability of your muscles and bones.

3. Stretching. This part is designed to help make you more flexible and supple.

THE BASIC RULES OF EXERCISE

BEFORE EMBARKING ON ANY EXERCISE PROGRAMME YOU SHOULD FOLLOW THESE EIGHT BASIC RULES

1. DO CONSULT YOUR DOCTOR BEFORE YOU BEGIN ANY EXERCISE PROGRAMME. IDEALLY YOU SHOULD ASK FOR A CHECK UP.

**2. DO TRAIN FOR A MINIMUM OF THREE AND A MAXIMUM OF

FIVE TIMES A WEEK. TRY TO TRAIN FOR BETWEEN 20 AND 60 MINUTES AT A TIME AND AIM AT A MINIMUM OF 60 MINUTES SOLID TRAINING EVERY WEEK, BUT NEVER DO MORE THAN 5 HOURS TRAINING IN ANY ONE WEEK.

3. ENSURE, WHENEVER POSSIBLE, THAT EACH INDIVIDUAL TRAINING SESSION INCLUDES ELEMENTS FROM EACH TYPE OF EXERCISE.

4. DO MAKE SURE THAT YOU WARM UP CAREFULLY BEFORE EVERY SESSION AND COOL DOWN CAREFULLY AFTER EVERY SESSION.

5. DO MAKE SURE THAT YOU AVOID ANYTHING THAT IS PAINFUL OR THAT YOU DO NOT ENJOY AND DO STOP IMMEDIATELY IF YOU GET A PAIN, SUFFER FROM BREATHLESSNESS, FEEL DIZZY OR NOTICE ANY OTHER SYMPTOMS.

6. VARY YOUR EXERCISE PROGRAMME CONSTANTLY IN ORDER TO MAINTAIN YOUR INTEREST AND TO MAXIMIZE YOUR GENERAL FITNESS LEVEL.

7. CONTINUE TO TRAIN REGULARLY EVEN WHEN YOU FEEL FIT, HEALTHY AND STRESS FREE.

8. IN ORDER TO GET THE BEST OUT OF YOUR EXERCISE PROGRAMME YOU SHOULD AIM TO GET AND TO KEEP YOUR PULSE RATE IN THE RANGE SHOWN OPPOSITE.

AGE	PULSE RANGE
15-19	120-180
20-24	115-175
25-29	115-170
30-34	110-165
35-39	105-160
40-44	105-155
45-49	100-150
50-54	95-145
55-59	95-140
60-64	90-135
65-69	90-135
70-74	80-130
75+	80-125

IMPROVING YOUR AEROBIC FITNESS

Some people equate fitness with physical strength, others mistake agility or skill for general fitness.

I regularly attend aerobics classes which I enjoy because they help me to stay fit and have fun, and help me to get rid of frustrations and aggressions and other manifestations of stress which build up during an ordinary working day.

Recently, a group of weight lifters and body builders, who were on holiday in the seaside town where I live, saw the notice advertising the aerobics class I attend and decided to join in.

From a conversation I overheard in the changing room beforehand, I rather gathered that for them the main attraction was the idea of working alongside twenty or thirty pretty young women dressed in tight fitting leotards. They certainly didn't imagine that they were going to have to work very hard. Like many people who have never tried an aerobics class, they thought that the class would be very easy.

When the class started the weight lifters and body builders, their huge muscles shining with oil, made rather loud and rude remarks about the simple warm up exercises the teacher was making us do before we got started. They were clearly unimpressed.

But after just ten minutes of the class the first of the bodybuilders gave up – exhausted. With sweat streaming off his body he had to go and sit on a wooden bench by the door. A few minutes later a second bodybuilder abandoned the class, complaining that he felt both out of breath and rather dizzy.

Not one of these huge and apparently super-fit men managed to last for more than half an hour, for the truth was that none of them were actually fit.

They were capable of lifting huge weights and they all had massive biceps and triceps muscles but they had done no aerobic work and their internal physical condition was poor.

In fact, this is by no means unusual among weight lifters and body builders. They specialize in building muscle bulk but they fail to put any effort at all into improving the condition of their hearts or lungs. Fitness – the capacity to do hard physical work without slowing down, weakening or getting tired – depends upon the condition of the whole body: the heart, the lungs an d the muscles. It really has nothing to do with agility.

In order to become truly fit you need to follow a balanced exercise programme and improving your aerobic fitness – the condition of your heart, your lungs and your muscles – is the first of the three important elements of a balanced programme.

Some people are reluctant to start a fitness programme because, they argue, their lives do not require them to be physically fit. They are wrong. We all need to be fit and we all benefit in many ways if we do make the effort to become physically fit. The human body was designed to be used and, like a machine, it works best when it is used regularly.

If you leave a car sitting in the garage for months at a time and you don't even start the engine occasionally, then you'll probably have difficulty in getting it to move when you finally need it, and you'll certainly find that it will behave sluggishly to begin with.

"A well-organized, regular exercise programme will help ensure you are less likely to suffer from dozens of different disorders."

The human body is the same. If you don't do any exercise at all, then your heart will grow weak, your muscles will become flabby and your whole body will become inefficient and less capable of coping with illness or pressure. Regular exercise helps to ensure that your body becomes better able to cope with emergencies of all kinds and more capable of resisting illness and infection. A well organized, regular exercise programme will help ensure that you are less likely to suffer from dozens of different disorders – including many types of back pain.

Other people argue that they feel unable to start any sort of exercise programme because they aren't fit enough. This, too, is wrong.

Everyone starting an exercise programme should, of course, get their doctor's approval before they start but even individuals who have become unfit can benefit from a well organized and regular exercise programme.

If you are not very fit you must remember that your exercise programme must start slowly and gently and then gradually build up as your fitness improves. The words 'gentle' and 'regular' are important, by the way. If you start an exhausting and over demanding exercise programme there is a real risk that you will injure yourself. And if you exercise only occasionally you will never become properly fit.

Study the aerobic choice table (opposite) and create your own personalized exercise programme. You should try to score at least 70 points a week to begin with – and then try to increase slowly to 100 points a week. You can measure out distances accurately by using a car or a bicycle fitted with a mileage indicator.

You will notice that the list of recommended exercises in the aerobic programme does not include things like isometrics (deliberately contracting muscles without producing movement) or callisthenics (exercises such as touching your toes which depend on flexibility, or press-ups which depend upon exisiting muscle strength); these exercises are not aerobic.

To build up your body's aerobic capacity you must exercise regularly and consistently in such a way that

AEROBIC EXERCISE CHOICE TABLE

1. RUNNING (OUT OF DOORS ON A FLAT COURSE OR ON A RUNNING MACHINE):

1 MILE IN 20 MINUTES OR LESS: 3 POINTS
1 MILE IN 15 MINUTES OR LESS: 6 POINTS
1 MILE IN 12 MINUTES OR LESS: 9 POINTS
1 MILE IN 10 MINUTES OR LESS: 12 POINTS
1 MILE IN 8 MINUTES OR LESS: 15 POINTS
IF YOU RUN FOR LONGER THAN 1 MILE, WORK OUT YOUR POINTS FROM YOUR TIME. SO, IF YOU COVER 2 MILES IN 20 MINUTES YOU GET 24 POINTS (FOR EXAMPLE, 2 X 1 MILE AT 10 MINUTES PER MILE OR 1 X 1 MILE AT 8 MINUTES PER MILE AND 1 X 1 MILE AT 12 MINUTES PER MILE).

NOTE: IF YOU ARE TOO TIRED TO KEEP RUNNING DON'T BE AFRAID TO STOP AND WALK. YOU CAN 'MIX AND MATCH' WALKING AND RUNNING AND STILL COLLECT POINTS.

---

2. WALKING (ON THE FLAT):

1 MILE IN 20 MINUTES OR LESS: 3 POINTS (NO POINTS IF WALKING SLOWER THAN 3 MPH UNLESS YOU WALK FOR MORE THAN AN HOUR – E.G. PLAYING GOLF – IN WHICH CASE YOU CAN SCORE 5 POINTS AN HOUR)

3. SWIMMING:

600 YARDS IN 15 MINUTES OR LESS: 15 POINTS

4. CYCLING (ON THE FLAT)
A) RACING BIKE:

2 MILES IN 12 MINUTES OR LESS: 3 POINTS
2 MILES IN 8 MINUTES OR LESS: 6 POINTS
2 MILES IN 6 MINUTES OR LESS: 9 POINTS
B) MOUNTAIN BIKE:
2 MILES IN 20 MINUTES OR LESS: 3 POINTS
2 MILES IN 14 MINUTES OR LESS: 6 POINTS
2 MILES IN 10 MINUTES OR LESS: 9 POINTS

5. SKIPPING:

10 MINUTES SKIPPING: 10 POINTS

6. AEROBICS CLASS:

A) BEGINNERS' CLASS:
60 MINUTES: 8 POINTS
B) INTERMEDIATE CLASS:
60 MINUTES: 10 POINTS
C) ADVANCED CLASS:
60 MINUTES: 15 POINTS

7. SQUASH, TENNIS, FOOTBALL, RUGBY, BASKETBALL ETC.
(ASSUMES MORE OR LESS CONTINUOUS EXERCISE – NO TIME ALLOWED FOR BREAKS ETC.):

60 MINUTES' PLAY: 15 POINTS

your lungs and heart have to start working more efficiently and more effectively in order to get oxygen supplies to your tissues, but you must take care not to over exercise. If you do too much aerobic training, there is a risk that you will put an excessive strain on your heart or that you will damage your joints.

Once so popular as a means of aerobic exercise, jogging has since gone out of fashion. Many enthusiasts ended up in hospital with back, hip, knee and ankle injuries caused by the hours and hours they spent pounding the streets.

The aim of the aerobic exercise programme is to improve your general fitness levels. It is not designed to turn you into an award-winning athelete. In order to build up your endurance levels, the exercise you choose must demand oxygen and must result in an increase in your heart rate. If your heart rate goes up to around 150 beats a minute (or to the upper end of the recommended aerobic range for your age) then your body will begin to benefit quite quickly – after about five minutes of exercise. If your heart rate doesn't go up quite that far, then you can still benefit, but you will have to exercise for longer.

RULES FOR AEROBIC EXERCISES

1. ALWAYS TALK TO YOUR DOCTOR FIRST ABOUT YOUR GENERAL HEALTH – AND GET HIS APPROVAL AND PERMISSION FOR YOUR EXERCISE PROGRAMME.

2. BEFORE AN EXERCISE SESSION YOU SHOULD MAKE SURE YOU LOOSEN YOUR JOINTS AND WARM UP YOUR MUSCLES AS WELL AS YOU CAN. IF YOU EXERCISE WITH COLD MUSCLES AND STIFF JOINTS YOU WILL INCREASE YOUR CHANCES OF ACQUIRING AN INJURY. SIMILARLY, IT IS IMPORTANT

THAT YOU COOL DOWN AFTER AN EXERCISE SESSION.

3. IF YOU EXERCISE EVERY DAY YOU WILL BECOME MENTALLY AND PHYSICALLY TIRED. SO TRY TO TAKE A REST DAY BETWEEN EXERCISE SESSIONS. TO GET THE BEST RESULT FROM YOUR EXERCISE PROGRAMME TRY TO EXERCISE THREE TIMES A WEEK.

4. YOU SHOULD BE SLIGHTLY OUT OF BREATH AND SWEATING A LITTLE BY THE MIDDLE OF A GOOD EXERCISE SESSION.

5. IF YOU ARE GOING TO BENEFIT FULLY AN EXERCISE SESSION SHOULD LAST AT LEAST TEN MINUTES AND PREFERABLY AT LEAST TWENTY MINUTES.

6. ALWAYS TALK TO A GOOD COACH BEFORE YOU START EXERCISING. MAKE SURE HE OR SHE KNOWS ABOUT MEDICAL CONDITION YOU MAY HAVE.

IMPROVING YOUR FLEXIBILITY

Many people who suffer from backache do so because their spines are stiff. Making your spine flexible will help you to reduce your chances of suffering from back trouble. Remember, there are dozens of joints in your spine and any one of them can cause pain and stiffness.

In addition to improving the flexibility of your spine you should also try to improve the flexibility of your other joints.

By spending a few minutes every week deliberately stretching and improving your flexibility you will help to improve your posture, make it easier for yourself to take part in the aerobic exercise sessions outlined above and reduce your chances of suffering from a wide range of muscle and joint disorders.

Remember, however, that you should never stretch in a way that you find painful; you should not 'bounce' when stretching (in an attempt to improve your reach) and you should be as gentle as possible.

IMPROVING YOUR STRENGTH

Until fairly recently I used to think that lifting weights and trying to build up muscles in the gym was a waste of time. Like many people I thought that lifting weights was only of value to vain and rather egotistical men who wanted to build up huge muscles so that they could show off on the beach.

But there is now evidence available to show that lifting weights can be of real value – and that weight training can play a vital part (though only a part!) in a complete exercise programme designed to increase your general fitness and to protect you against infirmity, disability and illness.

There is, I am delighted to say, even evidence available to show that weight training can help you however old you are!

Many old people fall down (and break bones and hazard their general health) because their muscles are weak but it is now agreed that a good, well organized weight training programme can help to improve muscle strength so effectively that falls become less likely.

An American research programme showed that after just two months of regular weight training exercises, a group of frail 90-year-old people who had never trained with weights before managed to double their muscle strength and, as a direct result, dramatically increase their ability to move about. Other researchers have shown that as well as increasing muscle strength and size, a properly coordinated weight lifting programme can actually help improve the strength of your bones! This means that if you do fall then you will be less likely to break a bone. Since many elderly people – and, in particular many backache sufferers – have 'thin' or 'frail' bones, weight lifting is clearly likely to offer a tremendous amount of protection.

Of course, you don't have to lift massive weights to benefit from this aspect of the fitness programme. And you certainly don't have to build up huge muscles! It isn't the size of the weights you lift that is important so much as the regularity with which you use them. As with so many other aspects of general fitness 'regular' is the key word!

STRENGTH ENHANCEMENT PROGRAMME

One of the big problems people face when they want to start lifting weights is finding somewhere suitable.

Some, older, more traditional gyms (the ones which specialize in helping enthusiastic body builders or weight lifters) can be, to the say least, a bit 'off putting' for most of us. However, these days, there is no shortage of suitable gyms to choose from. Most towns have at least one good, ordinary gym where people just wanting to 'keep fit' can work out. The important thing is that the equipment should be well maintained and in good condition and that there should be an expert advisor on hand who can tell you exactly how best to use the equipment!

Finally, do remember the golden rule: when using weights (as with every other form of exercise) you should never do anything at all that hurts. On the contrary you should always try to make sure that the exercise you do is fun!

TO INCREASE THE FLEXIBILITY OF YOUR LOWER BACK AND HAMSTRING MUSCLES

SIT ON THE FLOOR WITH YOUR LEGS STRAIGHT, YOUR KNEES LOCKED AND YOUR FEET TOUCHING A WALL. REST YOUR HANDS ON YOUR KNEES. SLOWLY BEND FORWARDS AND TRY TO TOUCH THE WALL. WHEN YOU HAVE REACHED AS FAR FORWARDS AS YOU CAN HOLD THE POSITION WHILE YOU COUNT UP TO FIVE. SIT BACK. RELAX WHILE YOU COUNT UP TO FIVE AND THEN REPEAT THE EXERCISE UP TO FIVE TIMES IF YOU CAN.

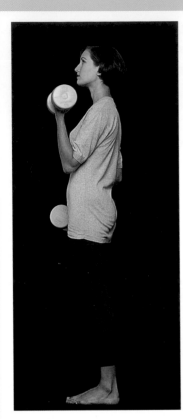

TO DEVELOP THE MUSCLES AT THE FRONT OF YOUR UPPER ARMS

1. *STAND WITH YOUR FEET SLIGHTLY APART HOLDING A DUMB-BELL IN EACH HAND. USING ONLY YOUR ARM MUSCLES LIFT THE RIGHT DUMB-BELL UP TO YOUR SHOULDER. THEN SLOWLY LOWER IT AGAIN. REPEAT THE EXERCISE WITH THE LEFT ARM.*

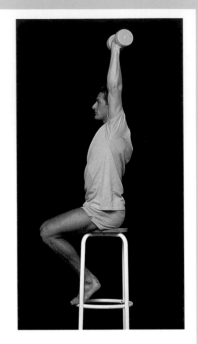

TO DEVELOP THE MUSCLES OF YOUR BACK, SHOULDERS AND THE BACKS OF YOUR UPPER ARMS

1. *SIT ON A CHAIR OR STOOL AND HOLD A DUMB-BELL IN EACH HAND AT SHOULDER HEIGHT. YOUR PALMS SHOULD BE FACING FORWARDS. PUSH YOUR RIGHT HAND UP UNTIL YOUR ARM IS FULLY EXTENDED. LOWER AND THEN REPEAT THE EXERCISE WITH YOUR LEFT HAND. LOWER AND THEN REPEAT THE EXERCISE.*

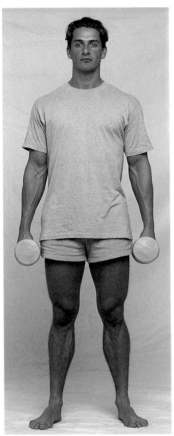

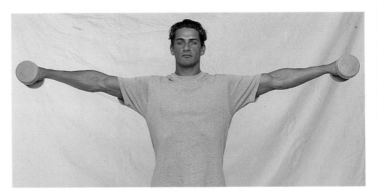

2. *STAND WITH YOUR FEET APART. YOUR HANDS, HOLDING YOUR DUMB-BELLS, SHOULD BE BY YOUR SIDES AND FACING INWARDS. THEN, MOVING BOTH ARMS AT ONCE, LIFT YOUR HANDS SIDEWAYS UNTIL YOUR ARMS ARE HORIZONTAL TO THE GROUND. LOWER AND THEN REPEAT THE EXERCISE.*

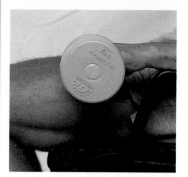

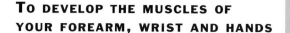

TO DEVELOP THE MUSCLES OF YOUR FOREARM, WRIST AND HANDS

1. SIT ON A CHAIR THAT HAS ARMS. REST YOUR FOREARMS ON THE ARM OF THE CHAIR WITH YOUR PALMS FACING DOWNWARDS. KEEP YOUR HAND AND WRIST OFF THE CHAIR ARM. ALLOW THE DUMB-BELL TO PULL YOUR HAND DOWNWARDS. LIFT THE DUMB-BELL IN YOUR RIGHT HAND BY USING YOUR WRIST. LOWER AND REPEAT THE EXERCISE WITH YOUR LEFT HAND. LOWER AND THEN REPEAT THE EXERCISE.

2. DO THE SAME EXERCISE WITH YOUR PALMS FACING UPWARDS.

WARNING
IT IS A MYTH THAT YOU NEED TO EXPERIENCE PAIN TO BENEFIT FROM EXERCISE. PAIN IS YOUR BODY'S WAY OF SAYING 'STOP'. IF YOU IGNORE A PAIN – OR TRY TO EXERCISE THROUGH IT – YOU WILL DO YOURSELF HARM.

TO DEVELOP THE MUSCLES AT THE SIDE OF YOUR BODY

1. STAND WITH YOUR FEET APART. HOLD A DUMB-BELL IN YOUR RIGHT HAND AND LET IT HANG AT ARM'S LENGTH. BEND TO THE RIGHT AS FAR AS YOU CAN. MOVE BACK TO THE UPRIGHT POSITION. BEND TO THE LEFT AS FAR AS YOU CAN. MOVE BACK TO THE UPRIGHT POSITION. SWAP THE DUMB-BELL TO YOUR OTHER HAND AND REPEAT THE EXERCISE.

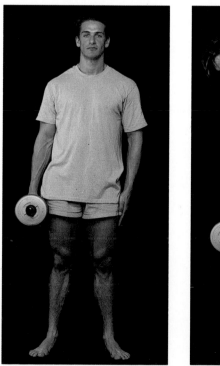

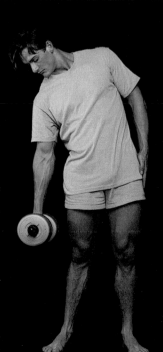

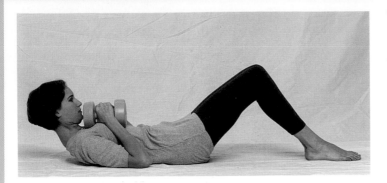

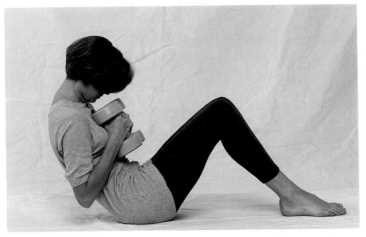

TO DEVELOP THE MUSCLES OF YOUR ABDOMEN

1. *LIE ON YOUR BACK WITH YOUR KNEES BENT AND YOUR FEET FLAT ON THE FLOOR. HOLD A DUMB-BELL ON YOUR CHEST WITH BOTH HANDS. TUCK YOUR CHIN INTO YOUR CHEST AND LIFT YOURSELF UP INTO A SITTING POSITION. LOWER YOURSELF SLOWLY. THEN REPEAT THE EXERCISE.*

TO DEVELOP THE MUSCLES OF YOUR THIGHS

1. *STAND WITH YOUR FEET APART HOLDING A DUMB-BELL IN EACH HAND WITH YOUR ARMS HANGING BY YOUR SIDES. KEEPING YOUR BACK STRAIGHT BEND YOUR KNEES UNTIL YOUR THIGHS ARE PARALLEL TO THE GROUND. RETURN TO THE STARTING POSITION AND THEN REPEAT THE EXERCISE.*

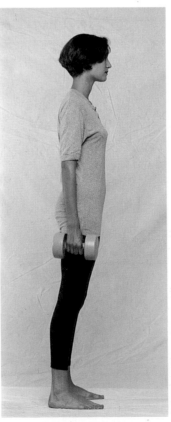

TO DEVELOP THE MUSCLES OF YOUR CALVES

1. STAND WITH YOUR TOES ON A THICK BOOK AND YOUR HEELS ON THE FLOOR. HOLD A DUMB-BELL IN EACH HAND WITH YOUR ARMS HANGING BY YOUR SIDES. LIFT YOUR HEELS OFF THE FLOOR AND THEN LOWER THEM BACK DOWN AGAIN. REPEAT THE EXERCISE.

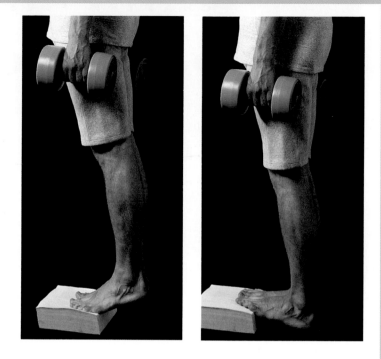

WARNING

IF YOU ATTEND AN AEROBICS CLASS MAKE SURE THAT IT IS 'LOW IMPACT AEROBICS' RATHER THAN 'HIGH IMPACT AEROBICS'. THE DIFFERENCE IS SIMPLE. IN 'LOW IMPACT AEROBICS' YOU ALWAYS KEEP ONE FOOT ON THE GROUND, WHEREAS IN 'HIGH IMPACT AEROBICS' THERE IS A LOT OF JUMPING AND LEAPING ABOUT WITH BOTH FEET IN THE AIR – AND AN INEVITABLE HEAVY IMPACT WHEN YOU LAND ON THE GROUND AGAIN.

THE RISK OF DEVELOPING A STRESS FRACTURE OR INJURING YOURSELF IN SOME OTHER WAY IS MUCH HIGHER WITH 'HIGH IMPACT AEROBICS'. ONE SURVEY OF 28 FITNESS CENTRES SHOWED THAT ONE IN TWO PEOPLE WHO ATTEND 'HIGH IMPACT AEROBICS' CLASSES INJURE THEMSELVES.

YOU CAN BUILD UP YOUR ENDURANCE LEVELS JUST AS WELL WITH 'LOW IMPACT AEROBICS' AS WITH 'HIGH IMPACT AEROBICS'.

MIX AND MATCH

To get more fun out of your aerobic exercise programme try as many different types of aerobic exercise as you can on different days of the week.

JOIN A GYM!

It is perfectly possible to get all the exercise you need in order to improve your physical fitness and help your mind conquer stress without ever going anywhere near a gym. But if there is a gym in your area I suggest that you join it! You'll benefit in a number of ways.

They are bound to have a wider range of equipment than you can buy for yourself and good gyms are staffed with well-qualified instructors who can help you develop an exercise programme to suit your own personal needs. You'll find, too, that most gyms are friendly places. You will benefit enormously from the support and companionship of those around you. It is much more fun and encouraging to exercise in a group than it is to exercise alone.

CHAPTER FIVE

What Doctors Can Do

Although it is always important to see your doctor if you are suffering from backache the majority of back pain sufferers will not get very much help from a physician or a surgeon. Most cases of backache are caused by strains and stresses for which there is no effective treatment apart from rest and painkillers.

There is little doubt that pain is the biggest single problem doctors have to face. Pain causes more unhappiness and more misery than all the other symptoms put together. The pain of a persistent and troublesome backache can ruin a career, a marriage and a life.

When pain is left untreated it can lead to physical and mental exhaustion, to disablement and to chronic anxiety. Patients with pain which is not treated properly are especially likely to develop medical complications. They are also likely to need additional medical treatment, and are likely to need to spend lengthy periods of time in hospital. People get better more slowly when they are in pain.

"Pain is the biggest single problem sufferers with back problems have to face."

Sadly, all the evidence seems to suggest that the majority of doctors are not very good at dealing with pain.

Speaking at the Third World Congress on Pain, one of the world's leading experts on pain relief pointed out that up to three-quarters of patients with persistent pain get poor treatment from their doctors. Other experts have made equally damning criticism of the medical profession. As one cynic put it, rather sadly, "Doctors are very good at tolerating other people's pain."

Medical schools spend very little time teaching students about pain or about pain relief, and a survey of medical text books showed that many did not discuss pain at all.

In a few cases, however, doctors *may* help. In this chapter I'm going to discuss the various things they can do.

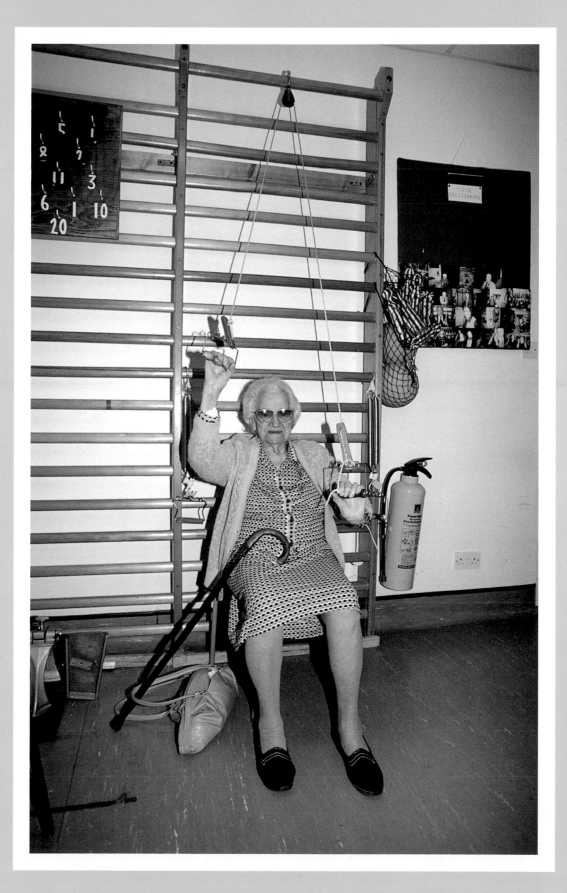

SURGERY

Although surgery can produce magnificent results in the treatment of prolapsed discs, fractured bones, compressed nerves and tumours, operations are often a last resort for backache and are only usually performed when other techniques have failed. (In a relatively small number of patients surgery is needed urgently, as an immediate solution, usually to prevent permanent damage to the spinal cord.)

Despite the fact that modern investigations enable surgeons to pinpoint problems with remarkable accuracy there are, inevitably, risks to be considered before surgery is contemplated. I suggest that you only accept a recommendation for surgery from a doctor whom you trust, and if a doctor recommends surgery you ask for a second opinion.

Any surgical operation involves risks: some patients react badly to an anaesthetic; there is always a risk of chest infection; bleeding can occur; and infections are always possible when tissues are opened up. In operating on the spine, however, surgeons know that they are taking especially large risks. The position and sensitivity of the spinal cord means that spinal surgery always includes a risk of paralysis.

Many patients who are in constant pain feel that the risks, which are much smaller these days than they used to be, are well worth taking, and there is no doubt that large numbers of people do benefit enormously after surgery. But few patients can report that all their pain is gone and those who expect a complete cure are usually disappointed. But a majority of patients do obtain some relief.

SPINAL FUSION

If your vertebrae are moving around too much or if a vertebra has slipped out of line your surgeon may recommend an operation called 'spinal fusion'. A slipping vertebra can result in pressure on the spine with resulting nerve pains, tingling and numbness.

The aim of the operation is to fix two or three vertebrae together permanently, and although the operation usually works well in removing nerve symptoms, the price that has to be paid is that part of the spine becomes rigid.

The fusion is normally done by taking a small piece of bone from another part of the body (usually the hip bone or pelvis, which can afford to lose a little piece of bone without being weakened or left deformed) which is used to make a graft to fix the vertebrae together. Sometimes the pieces of bone are fixed across the vertebrae which are to be joined, and sometimes the intervertebral disc is removed and replaced by the pieces of bone. Some surgeons use wire, rods and screws to fix the vertebrae together. The incision for the operation is usually made in the back but the operation can be done from the side or through the abdomen.

If you need a 'spinal fusion' operation you will probably be kept in bed for at least two or three weeks and then required to wear either a plaster cast or a surgical corset for another two months while the bones start to fuse together properly. It will take up to a year for the bone fusion to be completed.

DECOMPRESSION SURGERY

If something such as a protruding intervertebral disc or a piece of bone presses into your spinal canal your spinal cord will be compressed and the nerve pains will probably be severe and incapacitating. A 'decompression' operation is performed to relieve the pressure, eradicate symptoms and remove the danger of further damage being done to the spinal cord.

The operation is fairly crude. The surgeon will make an incision in your back and then simply chip away small bits of bone in order to make your spinal canal larger. If the bone is chipped away from the part of the vertebra called the lamina the operation is known as a laminectomy. However, if the bone is taken from the part of the vertebra known as the facet the operation is called a facetectomy.

If you need a 'spinal decompression' operation you should be able to go home within a week or so, but you will probably be told to avoid any heavy exercise for at least three months to give your body a chance to recuperate properly.

DISCECTOMY

This operation – which is a fairly common and relatively straightforward one – is performed when an intervertebral disc, or part of an intervertebral disc, has prolapsed (or 'slipped') and is pressing on a nerve and showing no signs of returning to its previous position.

If you need this operation your surgeon will usually remove just the part of the disc that is sticking out and causing the trouble, but if he feels that the remainder of the disc is likely to cause future problems by prolapsing again he may remove the whole of the disc nucleus.

In the traditional operation used for a discectomy the surgeon makes a fairly large incision in the patient's back, but these days a growing number of surgeons are performing this operation through a 1-inch long incision with the aid of a microscope.

Most patients get fairly immediate relief from pain if this operation is performed successfully and will be allowed up and about after two or three days and home after a week or so. However, heavy lifting or exercise will be banned for at least three months and many surgeons like their patients to wear a supportive corset for a few weeks after the operation.

PHYSIOTHERAPY

Physiotherapists use exercise, massage and manipulation to help patients, and because there are fewer risks involved most doctors prefer the majority of their patients to try physiotherapy before they consider surgery. As physiotherapy can produce a permanent improvement and long-term strengthening of the muscles it is usually also better than drug treatment – which is frequently aimed simply at relieving pain.

Most physiotherapists prefer to have access to X-rays and all the other investigations that have been ordered by doctors but they do also assess patients themselves and plan their treatment plan according to their conclusions. Physiotherapists' most important diagnostic aid is also their most important treatment aid – their hands – and they will learn most about you by touching and testing your muscles and back in general. He or she will, however, almost certainly also want to see you walk, sit and move in order to assess your posture and to spot any physical limitations.

MASSAGE, MANIPULATION AND MOBILIZATION

You don't need a physiotherapist to have a massage (see page 89) but the chances are that the massage you'll get from someone who is properly trained will do you far more good than the massage you'll get from a friend. A professional masseur will try to increase the mobility of your muscles and joints as well as break up toughened, fibrous tissue and improve poor blood supply. By stroking, kneading and stretching skin, muscles and other tissues the physiotherapist will be able to relax your muscles and take much of the stress and strain out of your back.

Manipulation techniques used by physiotherapists are identical to the ones used by osteopaths and chiropractors. A skilled manipulator will use his hands to move individual vertebrae and to unlock joints that have become fixed or restricted. Manipulative techniques can help rid muscle spasm, joint stiffness and many different varieties of back pain. It is obviously important that damaged joints and bones are not manipulated because in unskilled hands manipulation could lead to permanent damage of the spinal cord. You should never allow anyone who is not properly trained and qualified to manipulate any part of your body. Patients with disorders such as arthritis, osteoporosis and ankylosing spondylitis will probably not be suitable for manipulation because of the inflammation in their bones and the amount of weakness that has been produced.

Mobilization is a technique designed to flex stiff joints and to increase the possible range of movements. A joint will be carefully moved in order to stretch its ligaments, though it is important that the movement should not be painful.

TRACTION

If you have ever been into an orthopaedic ward in a hospital you will have almost certainly seen plenty of patients in traction, with their legs or arms suspended on the end of a complex-looking series of wires, pulleys and weights.

The aim when using traction for the treatment of patients with back trouble is usually to pull the joints of the back apart in order to release trapped nerves and to allow pieces of prolapsed disc to get back into the right position by taking the pressure off them. Normally, whenever you stand up the bones of your spine will be pushed closer and closer together, inevitably compressing any nerve that is trapped. Traction reverses that

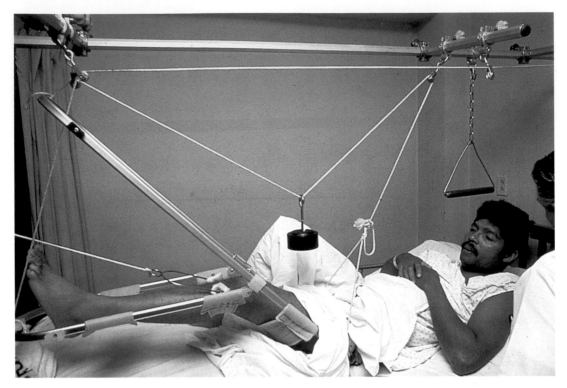

Traction is performed by means of a steel stirrup attached to the leg and pulled by weights

process. In addition to relieving pain, traction will often work to speed up the rate at which a patient makes a full recovery.

Traction has been used for thousands of years and it is basically very simple. Traditionally, patients with severe problems caused by disc protrusions were kept in continuous traction in hospital beds (though some doctors admit that this very simple technique was probably not a lot better than complete bed rest which allows the spine to stretch gently and naturally by itself), but today there are many variations available on this theme, and there are numerous different devices which will enable you to get the benefits of traction. Your physiotherapist may want to strap you to a table that swings you upside down or to a frame that enables you to control the amount of traction your spine is under yourself. (Beware of devices which send you upside down if you suffer from high blood pressure or eye problems or you have had a stroke in the past.) There are special halters for neck traction and you can even buy devices to help you hang from your door-frame so that the weight of your legs pulls on your back.

If you try traction and it causes you *more* pain tell

your physiotherapist immediately. He or she will almost certainly want to stop it straight away. Traction doesn't work for all patients.

ULTRASOUND

Ultrasound consists of high-frequency sound waves and is used as both a diagnostic and a treatment aid. It helps doctors make a diagnosis by showing up soft tissues which aren't clearly pictured on X-rays, and it is used by physiotherapists to help treat injuries to muscles, ligaments and joints by reducing inflammation, increasing blood flow and speeding up natural healing. A usual course of ultrasound lasts several weeks and consists of two or three sessions a week.

There are relatively few hazards with ultrasound (although it can cause bleeding if directed onto damaged tissues, it should be used with great caution on pregnant women and it can cause pain if directed onto a bone), and the only obvious consequences are usually a warm feeling and a certain amount of tingling.

If you feel ultrasound would benefit you then ask your doctor whether he thinks the treatment would help, and to recommend a physiotherapist.

TRANSCUTANEOUS NERVE STIMULATION

The devices used to apply this treatment are usually known as TENS machines and are described on page 84 in Chapter Six, since although they are commonly used by physiotherapists they can be bought or hired for use at home.

SHORT-WAVE DIATHERMY

This technique uses high-frequency electromagnetic waves which produce heat within the tissues. Different types of treatment affect tissues at different depths. The aim is to reduce swelling, increase blood flow and speed up the natural healing process. The procedure is painless and, like ultrasound, a course usually consists of two or three treatments a week for several weeks. Those who use short-wave diathermy usually claim that there are no known side effects.

INTERFERENTIAL THERAPY

Interferential therapy is another electrical treatment. Electrodes are attached to the skin where the pain is worst and the aim is to block the reception of pain impulses, to reduce the amount of inflammation and to improve the local circulation. It is also claimed that this technique can be used to help speed up the rate at which bone fractures heal.

Interferential therapy is usually given two or three times a week for several weeks, though some experts claim that it probably only provides short-term pain relief and may do relatively little to help speed up a long-term recovery.

CORSETS AND COLLARS

A back (or neck) that is sore or painful will often hurt less if some temporary support is provided by a fairly stiff corset or collar. There is a huge range of corsets and collars available – made from a variety of materials including canvas, foam, elastic and synthetic substances – and it is important that if you wear one it should fit you properly. Sometimes collars and corsets can be taken 'off the peg' but often they need to be specially tailored to fit.

In addition to providing some support, corsets and collars also help by stimulating nerve endings (and sup-

pressing some pain impulses), keeping the area warm (heat helps to relieve pain) and by preventing sudden and potentially excruciating movements.

Corsets and collars are usually short-term solutions and are probably not suitable for long-term use since they can, if used for long periods, result in the spine becoming stiff.

INJECTIONS

There are several different ways in which doctors can inject drugs into your back in order to try to relieve pain, stiffness and discomfort. Some doctors are very enthusiastic about injections, others feel that they are over-rated and that the hazards make them unsuitable for general use. I recommend that you only accept an injection from a doctor that you trust and that you always try to get a second opinion before having anything injected into your spine.

STEROID INJECTIONS

Local injections of corticosteroid are frequently used to combat specific muscle pains and to help increase the rate at which a sprained ligament heals. Steroids do relieve pain and inflammation, but there can be serious problems if they are used too often or in large quantities. Because steroids are natural hormones, produced within your body to help combat all types of injury and inflammation, one of the main dangers is that over-use of steroids could suppress your body's own production of steroids – which could make you vulnerable to disease and infection. Long-term steroid use can also lead to weight gain, acne, excessive hair growth, high blood pressure, diabetes and osteoporosis.

Having said all that, it is true that steroid injections are almost certainly safer than steroids taken by mouth. Steroids given by injection can be given in fairly small, controlled doses and can be applied directly to the area needing treatment. Steroids given by mouth are much more of a 'blunderbuss' therapy.

SCLEROSING INJECTIONS (PROLOTHERAPY)

A sclerosant injection contains an irritant which stimulates the production of new fibrous tissue and new collagen. These injections are given directly into ligaments which help to hold together joints and which need to be tightened or made stronger. After a series of sclerosing injections there will first be a feeling of bruising and then, after about two months, enough ligament tissue will have grown to strengthen the joint.

EPIDURAL INJECTIONS

Patients who have severe back pain and who have a damaged nerve – with weak muscles and numb areas of skin – may benefit if an anaesthetic injection is given into the epidural space in the spine. This type of injection seems particularly useful for patients who have prolapsed discs producing nerve pain that has not responded to any other sort of treatment.

The injection is given into the space between the bony outer walls of the spinal canal and the membrane which covers the spinal cord, and in addition to containing an anaesthetic the injection usually contains a steroid. The anaesthetic numbs the spinal cord and the steroid helps to reduce the amount of local inflammation which has been caused by the prolapsed disc.

The pain relief produced by an epidural injection may be temporary or permanent, and about half of all patients get at least some relief. The procedure is fairly uncomfortable but the relief can be tremendous.

CHYMOPAPAIN INJECTION

Chymopapain is an enzyme derived from the papaya fruit and it digests protein. When injected directly into a prolapsed intervertebral disc it dissolves the soft central nucleus of the disc. As the nucleus dissolves so the disc shrinks and the pressure on whatever is trapped will be relieved. There is a considerable amount of controversy about this treatment, but some doctors feel that it is safer than surgery – and more helpful. The technique is probably less likely to produce complications than it was when first introduced some years ago.

DRUGS ON PRESCRIPTION

With the exception of steroids (which can produce a magical effect but which demand a high potential price in side effects) the only really useful drugs available for the treatment of back trouble are painkillers. Sadly, there are no entirely safe pills that you can take which will 'cure' a prolapsed disc or 'heal' a stiff joint, although some painkillers do also have an anti-inflammatory effect which may help increase the rate at which a back problem gets better. By and large pills prescribed for back pain will not treat the cause of the trouble but merely help to soothe the symptoms.

The corticosteroids are a group of drugs which are similar to the natural corticosteroid hormones produced by the adrenal glands. They are used in a wide variety of inflammatory disorders (including many different types of arthritis) and when injected into inflamed tendons or joints can relieve pain and stiffness. Although the corticosteroids are extremely effective they do produce a wide variety of serious side effects – particularly if used for long periods and in high dosages. (See steroid injections.)

For most people drugs are still the most common way of dealing with pain – and there are scores, if not hundreds, of apparently different painkillers available. However, 99 per cent of all drugs used as painkillers come either from the willow tree or poppy families: aspirin and morphine (the opiates).

THE ASPIRIN FAMILY

The effectiveness of acetylsalicylic acid (the drug extracted from the willow) was first described in a scientific paper some 200 years ago, but it wasn't until the end of the 19th century that tablets called 'aspirin' first came onto the market and were made readily available in chemists' shops.

The salicylates may be the most popular drugs to have come from the willow tree, but during the last few decades chemists have taken many more products from the same basic source. Drugs such as phenylbutazone, paracetamol, indomethacin, mefanamic acid and ibuprofen all come from the same plant.

Although we still don't really know exactly how any of these drugs work we do know that they suppress inflammation, pain and fever with varying degrees of effectiveness – and with varying side effects. One possible explanation is that drugs such as aspirin block the synthesis of prostaglandins, the chemicals which the

The willow tree is the source of many pain-killing drugs such as aspirin

76

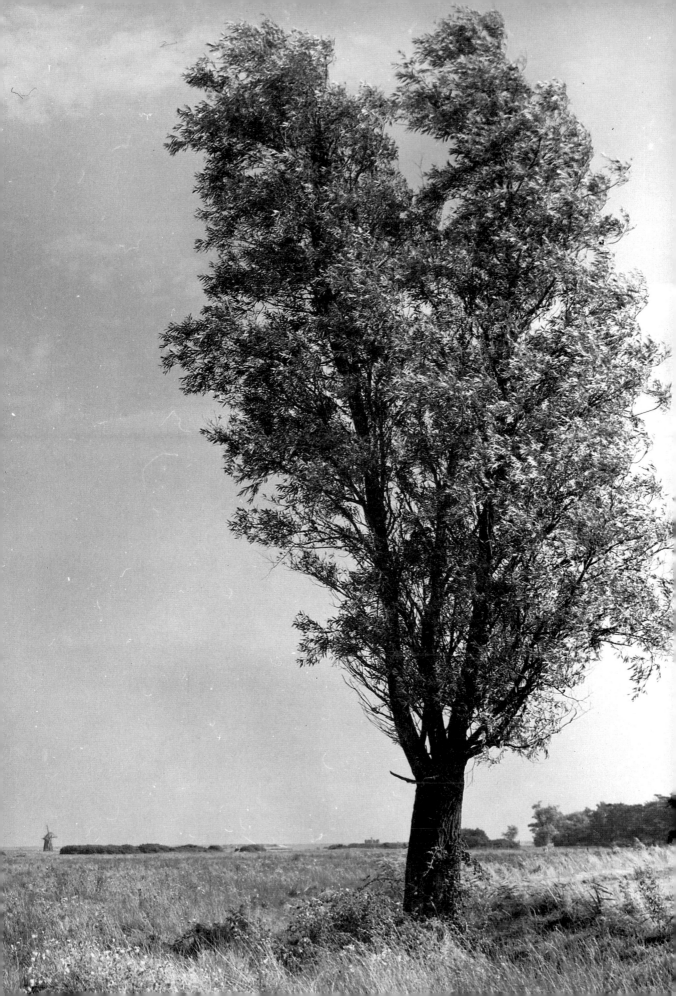

body produces when bodily tissues are damaged and which are responsible for producing swelling around the site of the injury and stimulating the nerve endings to send pain messages travelling up to the brain.

Aspirin and all the other drugs in this group can cause a number of side effects. The most common problem associated with aspirin is probably gastric irritation and bleeding, but patients who take too many aspirin tablets are also likely to complain of dizziness and ringing in their ears. There are some patients who are sensitive to all the products in this group and cannot take any of them without feeling uncomfortable or developing unpleasant and potentially dangerous allergy symptoms.

"Although we still don't really know exactly how any of these drugs work we do know that they suppress inflamation, pain and fever..."

The existence of these side effects has, however, been over-emphasized in the last few years. Aspirin tablets can prove lethal but in my view the dangers have probably been exaggerated by drug companies anxious to sell alternative products. Since there are so many companies manufacturing versions of aspirin the price is low and the profits limited.

Partly because aspirin is made and sold in so many forms drug companies have produced their own brands of painkillers. So, for sale directly over the chemists' counter are now many products containing a mixture of one or more ingredients from aspirin, paracetamol, caffeine and codeine.

The one really useful advance that has been made has involved the development of soluble aspirin tablets which can be swallowed in liquid form rather than as tablets. Soluble aspirin tablets are far less likely to cause stomach irritation and are, therefore, safer than the ordinary old-fashioned, non-soluble type.

Because doctors are slightly more difficult to dupe than ordinary customers, the drug companies have been more sophisticated in their attempts to introduce new prescription-only painkillers to replace aspirin tablets, using all sorts of clever tricks to convince them of the value of the latest product. One trick has been to produce a new 'alternative' drug and then to measure its effectiveness – and the likelihood of side effects

being produced – against that of ordinary, insoluble aspirin: this means it isn't too difficult to show that the new product is less dangerous. But if the product had been compared to soluble aspirin then the results might have been less flattering.

During the last 20 years or so an extraordinary number of alternative painkillers have been launched. Many have been specifically designed for use by those suffering from backache and arthritis – both problems which affect millions of patients and which tend to persist for many years (criteria which make a drug especially profitable to the drug companies). Many of these drugs have been promoted for their anti-inflammatory properties as much as for their painkilling properties.

Sadly, some of these aspirin alternatives have lasted only a year or two before having to be removed from the market because of unpleasant side effects; others have remained on the market despite a lack of any really convincing, independent evidence to show that they are superior to aspirin.

THE OPIATE FAMILY

The history of the opiates – drugs originally extracted from the opium poppy – goes back several thousand years, and both Hippocrates and the great Roman physician, Galen, used to prescribe opium for reliving pain. By the 19th century opium had become probably the most popular drug in the world and it was widely used throughout Europe. During the so-called 'Opium Wars' the British fought the Chinese for the right to continue exporting opium to China and in the single year of 1870 no less than 90,000 lb of opium were officially and legally imported into Britain.

There are as many variations on the opium theme as there are on the aspirin theme. Opium contains about 10 per cent morphine and rather smaller amounts of other substances (including codeine), and from these basic constituents a number of products have been prepared for the treatment of pain. All tend to provide a considerable amount of pain relief but make the people who take them feel sleepy.

Although the opiates have been used as effective painkillers for thousands of years it has only been fairly recently that doctors have managed to work out exactly how they work. It seems that morphine, heroin and the other opiates imitate natural hormones – called endorphins and enkephalins – which are produced within the brain as the body's own special answers to pain. These hormones can switch off the body's pain alarm by fitting into special receptors on nerve cells.

Your body needs these internal pain relieving hormones when it needs to overcome pain in order to survive. For example, if you had injured your ankle but needed to keep running in order to save your life your body would numb the pain of the damaged ankle with its internally produced endorphins so that you would be able to ignore the pain and keep on running. Those same endorphins are also produced when you are busy and doing something that your mind thinks is more important than pain. So, for example, if you are playing in an important golf, tennis or football match and you strain a muscle that would normally stop you moving, your body will produce endorphins so that you can ignore the pain and carry on playing. Only when the match is over will the endorphin production stop – then you will feel the pain.

Morphine, heroin and other drugs we think of as powerful painkillers are, in fact, really nothing more than counterfeit endorphins. They achieve their effect by interacting with those natural receptors and by imitating the effect of your body's own natural, pain relieving hormones.

Because the opiates also have an effect on the mood of the person taking them these drugs have, in recent years, been involved in a great deal of controversy, and some patients are wary of taking them in case they become addicted. However, the evidence shows quite conclusively that it is extremely rare for patients who use opiates to relieve pain to become addicted. In a survey made of thousands of Israeli casualties in the Yom Kippur War in 1973 it was found that although many of the wounded soldiers had been given morphine not one of them had become addicted to it. Similar evidence was produced by American doctors working with soldiers wounded in Vietnam.

TRANQUILLIZERS

Many doctors prescribe benzodiazepine tranquillizers for patients suffering from back pain on the grounds that these drugs help to relieve tension, anxiety and stress and will, therefore, help to overcome muscle tension and muscle spasms. Because the benzodiazepines also help to make patients feel sleepy they are frequently prescribed for patients whose pain prevents them from getting to sleep at night.

However, in addition to producing a variety of unpleasant side effects (after being taken for a few weeks the benzodiazepines can make a patient feel anxious and depressed and can themselves produce insomnia), these drugs are now known to be potentially very addictive. Some researchers also believe that drugs in the benzodiazepine group can make some patients *more* sensitive to pain.

Most experts now agree that because of these problems (particularly the risk of addiction) these drugs should not be prescribed for more than two weeks at a time. Since back pain is often a long-term problem, that constraint alone makes the benzodiazepines unsuitable for back pain sufferers.

GETTING THE BEST
OUT OF DRUGS

Drugs are not always used wisely or effectively. One recent survey of 800 patients who had been given drugs for pain relief showed that 14 per cent had given up taking the drugs that had been prescribed for them because they felt that they were not deriving any benefit from them. An even larger group who were still taking their drugs claimed that they were deriving no benefit from them at all.

One of the reasons for the failure of powerful drugs to provide patients with any useful relief is undoubtedly the fact that many doctors who prescribe these substances do not understand how best they can be used. If you are going to take drugs to control your pain, you would be wise to understand a little about how drugs work.

There are really only three drugs for the treatment of pain: aspirin, codeine and morphine. There are hundreds of alternatives to these three basic drugs but I have not seen any evidence to show that any of these alternatives are better than these products. Those patients who cannot take aspirin because they are sensitive to it can substitute paracetamol, but otherwise there is little point in trying variations on these themes. Aspirin is the weakest of these drugs and morphine the most powerful. Codeine provides a level of pain relief somewhere in between the two.

If a pain cannot be relieved by ordinary soluble aspirin then it is probably more sensible to increase the dose than to switch to an alternative but basically similar product. If the pain has not been effectively controlled when the maximum permitted dose of aspirin has been reached then the sensible move is to change either to codeine or directly to morphine.

When taking a painkiller it is important to take the drug in a large enough quantity. One of the main reasons why so many people fail to get proper relief from the drugs they take is that they are not taking them in large enough doses. Many patients, both in home and in hospital, receive only one-quarter of the dose they need to control their pain. And both doctors and nurses frequently underestimate the extent of patients' pain, overestimate the power of the drugs they use, and worry far too much about the danger of their patients becoming addicted.

"Even in these days of apparently high-technology medicine there are many variations in the treatments preferred by differing doctors."

If you are going to take a drug there is no point in taking it unless you get proper pain relief. If the drug you are taking does not help then ask your doctor to increase the dosage.

It is also important to take your painkiller regularly. You should not wait until your pain returns before taking the next dose of pills. This is not a sign of strength but one of ignorance. By taking a drug only when you are in terrible pain you will be weakening your body, and by learning to associate your drug with relief from pain, you will be making yourself more dependent on drug relief than you would be if you took your pills at regular times.

Painkilling drugs should be taken according to the clock and not according to the presence or absence of pain. If this philosophy is followed then it will be possible to keep the amount of painkilling drug that you need to an absolute minimum.

A WARNING ABOUT DOCTORS

When you go to the doctor for help and treatment you probably assume that once they have decided what is wrong with you they will automatically give you a treatment that is quite specific for your disease.

Nothing could be further from the truth.

With a very few exceptions there are no certainties in medicine. What you get will depend more on chance and your doctor's personal prejudices than on science.

This problem isn't a new one, of course. In the preface to *The Doctor's Dilemma*, playwright George Bernard Shaw points out that during the first great epidemic of influenza which developed towards the end of the 19th century, a London evening newspaper sent a journalist posing as a patient to all the great consultants of the day. The newspaper then published details of the advice and prescriptions offered by the consultants. The whole proceeding was, almost inevitably, passionately denounced by the medical journals as an unforgivable breach of confidence, but the result was fascinating nevertheless: despite the fact that the journalist had complained of exactly the same symptoms to the many different physicians, the advice and the prescriptions that were offered were all different.

Nothing has changed. Even in these days of apparently high-technology medicine there are many – almost endless – variations in the treatments preferred by differing doctors.

Doctors offer different prescriptions for exactly the same symptoms; they keep patients in hospital for vastly different lengths of time for the same illness, and they perform different operations on patients with apparently identical problems.

There are, it seems, no certainties in medicine.

The unexpected seems to happen so often that it

really ought to be expected, and the likelihood of a doctor accurately predicting the outcome of a disease is often no more than 50:50. (After carrying out 400 post-mortem examinations two pathologists reported recently that they had found that in more than half the patients the wrong diagnosis had been made.)

There is, indeed, ample evidence now available to show that the type of treatment a patient will get when he visits his general practitioner will depend not so much on the symptoms he describes but on the doctor he consults.

So, for example, consider what happened when 430 Scottish family doctors were asked to explain how they would treat a 35-year-old accountant complaining of backache brought on by digging in his garden. The 'case history' was deliberately made fairly precise, but despite this precision the treatments recommended by each doctor varied enormously.

Less than one-quarter of the doctors said that they would definitely prescribe a painkiller. Nearly 10 per cent said that they hardly ever prescribed a painkiller in such circumstances. Eight per cent said they might refer the patient to hospital but 52 per cent said that they never referred such patients to hospital. Forty-eight per cent said that they usually advised bed rest for up to one week while 8 per cent said that they usually advised bed rest for between one and four weeks. Around 10 per cent of the doctors said that there was a good chance that they would refer the patient to an osteopath but the other 90 per cent said that they hardly ever, or never, referred patients to osteopaths. Such enormous differences in opinion are surprisingly commonplace these days.

Going to your family doctor really is, it seems, something of a lottery!

Despite all these variations in the type of treatment offered most doctors in practice seem convinced that their treatment methods are beyond question. Many GPs and hospital doctors announce their decisions as though they are carved on stone.

On the basis of the evidence, however, it seems that most decisions about how patients should be treated for common ailments are based on nothing more scientific than guesswork, personal experience, intuition and prejudice.

HOW TO USE DRUGS WISELY

1. IF YOU TAKE DRUGS REGULARLY YOU SHOULD TAKE THEM AT FIXED TIMES AND YOU SHOULD *NOT* WAIT UNTIL YOUR PAIN RETURNS.

2. *DO NOT TAKE MORE THAN ONE LOT OF DRUGS AT ONCE UNLESS YOUR DOCTOR HAS SPECIFICALLY INSTRUCTED YOU TO DO SO AND KNOWS WHAT YOU ARE TAKING. NOT ALL DRUGS MIX WELL.*

3. DRUGS SHOULD ONLY EVER PLAY A *PART* IN YOUR PAIN CONTROL PROGRAMME.

4. *REMEMBER THAT PAINKILLING DRUGS CAN ONLY EVER MASK A CONDITION – THEY CANNOT CURE IT.*

5. ALWAYS TRY TO TAKE THE SMALLEST DOSE POSSIBLE TO CONTROL YOUR PAIN. IF YOU WANT TO CUT DOWN YOUR CONSUMPTION OF DRUGS TALK TO YOUR DOCTOR FIRST. IT IS USUALLY BETTER TO CUT DOWN THE DOSAGE YOU TAKE RATHER THAN THE NUMBER OF TIMES A DAY THAT YOU TAKE YOUR DRUG. FOR EXAMPLE, IF YOU TAKE THREE ASPIRIN TABLETS FOUR TIMES A DAY TRY TO CUT DOWN TO TWO TABLETS FOUR TIMES A DAY RATHER THAN THREE TABLETS THREE TIMES A DAY.

6. *IF YOU NOTICE ANY SIDE EFFECTS OR UNEXPECTED SYMPTOMS WHILE TAKING A DRUG ALWAYS TELL YOUR DOCTOR AND ASK HIS ADVICE.*

CHAPTER SIX

Controlling The Pain

Pain is the biggest single problem sufferers with back problems have to face. It causes more misery, more unhappiness and more despair than all other symptoms put together. It ruins the lives of millions and wrecks careers and relationships. When left untreated or badly treated, pain may lead to physical and mental exhaustion, disablement and chronic depression. Patients with persistent pain need to spend long periods in bed and are far more likely to develop other serious medical complications. Patients with pain get better more slowly and need more support from friends, family and professionals.

Despite all this, pain is usually treated badly by the professionals and at least three-quarters of all patients with persistent back pain get poor treatment from their doctors.

"Pain causes more unhappiness and more misery than all the other symptoms put together"

There are several reasons for this but the most important one is undoubtedly the fact that medical schools spend very little time teaching students about pain or about pain relief. A recent survey of 17 standard medical textbooks found that out of 22,000 pages only 54 provided any information at all about pain! Half the standard textbooks used by medical students and doctors do not discuss pain at all.

The result is that many doctors tell patients who are suffering from pain simply to 'take things easy' or to 'grit their teeth and be brave' and too often they simply turn to drug treatment as a first line of attack.

For many years researchers have been searching for, identifying and testing new ways of dealing with pain. Many of the techniques they have discovered are safe, effective and inexpensive. But the drug companies have no interest in non-drug therapies and so the majority of practising doctors, who get much of their education from drug company sponsored literature, continue to ignore these treatments.

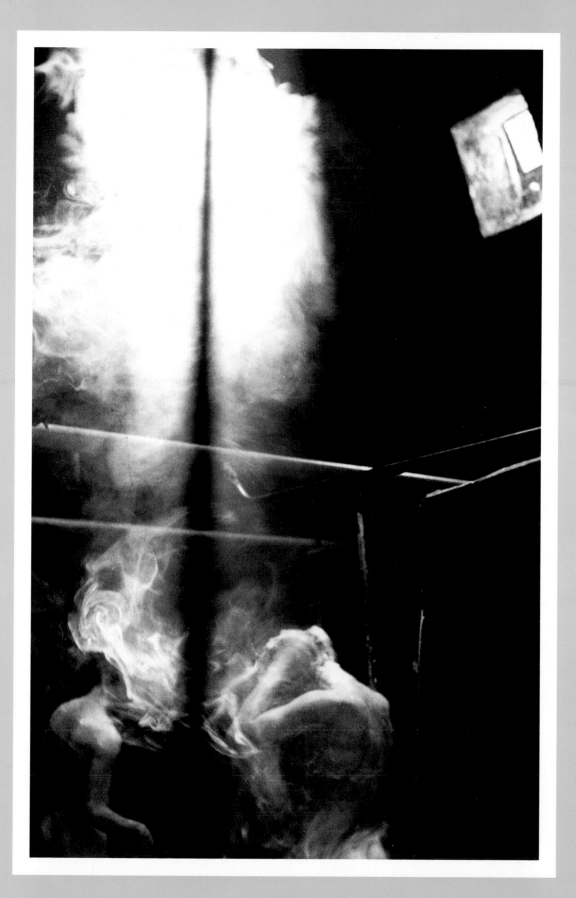

How To Measure Your Pain

It is impossible to measure pain objectively. There are so many different factors involved that it is hard for you to compare the pain you get in your back with the pain your neighbour gets in her womb. But you can measure variations in a particular pain and tell whether or not a specific pain is getting better or worse. By doing so you can work out whether or not a pain relieving technique that you are using is working.

Next time you want to measure your pain look through the list again and repeat the procedure, comparing your total score with previous total scores.

TENS MACHINES

A Transcutaneous Electrical Nerve Stimulation machine is a remarkable device which can help remove backache extremely effectively at very low cost and with few side effects. To understand how it works I must explain a little about how your body recognizes pain.

The gate control theory of pain put forward by two scientists called Melzack and Wall suggested that when body tissues are damaged messages carrying information about the injury travel towards the brain along two quite separate sets of nerve fibres. The larger fibres carry messages about sensations other than pain, and the smaller fibres carry the pain messages. The messages which travel along the larger fibres tend to arrive at the spinal cord before the messages travelling along the smaller fibres and, if there are enough non painful sensations travelling, the pain messages won't be able to get through to the brain.

Once this theory had been accepted it was possible to explain all sorts of natural phenomena which had, up until then, been a mystery.

So, for example, it became clear that when we rub a sore spot what we are doing is increasing the number of non-pain messages travelling towards the spinal cord (and thence the brain). If you knock your elbow you will automatically reach to rub the spot because subconsciously you know that by rubbing the area you will be able to cut down the amount of pain that you feel.

Having realized just how rubbing a sore or painful place can relieve pain, the next step for scientists was to come up with a way of stimulating the passage of non-painful sensations even more efficiently. Doctors came up with the idea of using electrical pulses to produce the necessary stimulus.

When the theory was first put into practice in the late 1960s doctors suggested that electricity should be introduced into the body through electrodes surgically implanted in the spine. Although that did work, the fact that it involved an operation limited the usefulness and availability of the procedure.

Next, it was discovered that all nerves within an

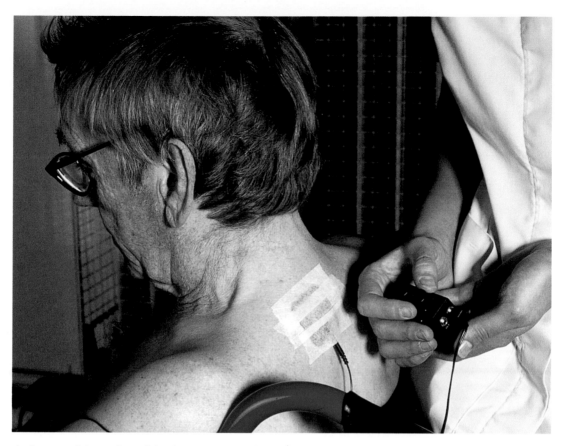

inch or so of the surface of the skin can be stimulated by electrodes which are simply stuck onto the skin. That encouraged medical researchers to start giving patients pocket-sized battery-operated stimulators which sent out a continuous series of electrical pulses which could transmit those pulses into the large nerves of the body via silicon electrodes stuck to the skin with a special conducting paste. It worked!

More exciting still, it was discovered that Transcutaneous Electrical Nerve Stimulation (it quickly became known as TENS) did not just stimulate the passage of sensory impulses designed to inhibit the passage of pain impulses; it also stimulated the body to start producing its own pain-relieving hormones known as endorphins.

During the last ten years an enormous number of research projects have shown that TENS machines are convenient, safe and effective. They are also cheap to buy and extremely cheap to run.

In a study of patients suffering from rheumatoid arthritis it was found that TENS equipment produced pain relief in up to 95 per cent of patients with up to

A TENS machine is fairly inexpensive, easy to use and usually free of unpleasant side effects

50 per cent of patients getting long-term relief.

But it isn't just arthritis patients who benefit from using TENS machines. According to Professor John Thompson of the University of Newcastle upon Tyne, England, (who is the consultant in charge of the pain relief clinic at the Royal Victoria Infirmary in Newcastle) up to 90 per cent of patients get short-term relief from pain and 35 per cent of patients are still benefiting after two years of use.

TENS machines have been shown to be effective in the treatment of all kinds of pain. For example, a Swedish study has shown that TENS machines are the only painkillers required by 70 per cent of women in labour; and backache is one of the types of pain best treated with TENS machines.

With this sort of success available from a small, cheap, portable, long-lasting machine that can be used at home without any training and that does not seem to produce any side effects at all, you might imagine that doctors would be recommending TENS machines to millions of patients and that shops would have different models stocked high on their shelves. But if you try to buy a TENS machine you'll have difficulty.

Why?

Because drug companies don't want patients in pain to be able to deal with their symptom so easily, quickly and cheaply. Drug companies make huge amounts of money out of selling painkillers to pain sufferers and if people used TENS machines instead it would cost them a fortune in lost sales.

You ought to be able to buy one at your chemist's. But I doubt if you'll be able to. However, there is some good news. If you want to try a TENS machine ask your doctor to refer you to the nearest pain clinic. You should be able to get one on loan and if you find that the machine works for you then you should be able to obtain one for permanent use.

(Using electricity to treat pain isn't new. The ancient Egyptians used electricity to treat pain, as did Hippocrates. One Roman physician cured headaches with the energy produced by electric torpedo fish. Another claimed that gout could be cured by putting the feet in a bucket of water along with an electric eel.)

THE VIBRATOR

Stroking and rubbing a sore area helps to control pain by stimulating the production of sensory nerve impulses which travel quickly along the larger nerve fibres, get to the gate in the spinal cord first and block the passageway of pain impulses. This is how the TENS machine works.

If you cannot afford a TENS device, or don't want to buy one, then you may be able to obtain a very similar effect by using a vibrator – exactly the same sort of hand-held vibrator as is sold in pharmacies and sex shops for 'personal massage'.

When an ordinary vibrator was used by 17 patients suffering from facial pain and held on the relevant area for 30 minutes, 14 of the patients reported that their pain was significantly reduced both during stimulation and for some time afterwards. Eight out of the 17 patients reported that they obtained relief for between four and six hours afterwards. These patients reported that the vibrator was more effective than anything else

they had tried. Most important of all, a year after the initial experiment the patients were still getting pain relief from their vibrators.

Another research project showed that 47 out of 50 patients obtained pain relief by using a vibrator.

Talk to your doctor and ask him if he thinks your pain could be helped in this way.

HEAT

Heat has been used to help relieve pain for centuries and just about every country in the world has a history of using spas, saunas, hot springs, baths and soaking tubs to help eradicate pain. Although heat can help just about any sort of pain it is particularly effective in the relief of backache.

Just how heat produces its useful effect is still something of a mystery although scientists have put forward several theories. It has been suggested that heat generates nerve impulses which help stop pain impulses getting through to the brain. Alternatively it may be that since it is the responsibility of the blood to remove products such as histamine and prostaglandins (chemicals which are produced by the body and which are responsible for the sensation of pain) and since heating the tissues increases the flow of blood, heating the body may increase the rate at which pain disappears.

The truth is that both these theories are probably correct, although to a certain extent the question of just how heat relieves pain is rather academic, since the important thing is that heat *does* relieve pain.

There are numerous ways of applying heat to your body. The best way is probably by having a warm bath. Millions of sportspeople and gardeners will confirm that nothing soothes sore and inflamed muscles quite as much as lying down in a bathful of warm water. As an alternative to an ordinary hot bath at home you could try visiting your nearest well-heated swimming pool, sauna or steam room.

If you want to apply heat to specific areas of your body then you can try using heated towels, an electrically heated pad, a sun lamp or an old-fashioned hot-water bottle. If you do try using a hot-water bottle do make sure that the rubber is not perished, that the stopper fits well and that the bottle is wrapped in a towel so that it does not burn your skin.

ICE

Even more surprising than heat as a treatment for backache is ice. Few of us think of ice as being a useful remedy for pain, but it is. Indeed, cold is often even more effective than heat at reducing backache.

A specialist at Boston Pain Clinic in the United States has claimed that after being massaged with ice many patients get up to four hours of pain relief. He reported that 78 per cent of his backache patients got significant pain relief.

How does ice work? I'm not sure that anyone really knows. One theory is that it constricts the blood vessels and makes the area feel numb. Another theory is that ice produces pain-relieving endorphins and interferes with the passage of pain impulses.

To avoid being cut by sharp-edged pieces of ice, put ice cubes into a rubber ice bag or hot-water bottle. Alternatively, you can simply wrap ice cubes in a thin cloth such as a tea towel.

Whatever you choose you can best get relief by rubbing the ice all over the painful area in circular or backwards and forwards movements. Press fairly firmly. When you rub ice on your skin you should first feel the cold, then feel a burning and then a stiffness. Finally there is a numbness. You should not hold the ice in contact with your skin for more than five minutes at a time – remember that ice, like heat, can burn. You should keep the ice moving so that it doesn't remain in contact with one part of the skin for more than a few seconds. As soon as your skin feels numb you should remove the ice and start to move the area immediately. You should notice that the whole area is more easily moveable quite quickly.

MUSIC

Most people enjoy music of some sort, from Beethoven to the latest chart success. Music can cheer you up when you are feeling sad or irritable; it can calm you down when you are feeling anxious or stressed; and it can help you overcome despair and depression.

But music can have a much more powerful effect. It can actually help in the healing process. Although the healing power of music was widely recognized in ancient times, it has only recently been used in modern medicine to help patients with both physical and mental illnesses. Nowadays there are trained music therapists who help patients recover by encouraging them to listen to and participate in music. Music can also be used as an effective way of communication and self-expression for mentally ill or disabled children and adults. It can penetrate and benefit the mind that is deaf to conversation. The power of music can even have a beneficial effect on the unconscious mind; patients in a coma benefit from hearing a favourite piece of music or song and playing a tape of pulsating sounds as a reminder of the womb helps ensure that premature babies stay alive.

A Scottish psychiatrist called Dr Isaac Sclare was the first to use soothing music to help patients recover from a wide range of mental disorders. Since his pioneering work it has been demonstrated that various forms of music can be used effectively in the treatment of mental and emotional problems, as well as to soothe and relieve pain.

Music is a very good way of keeping your mind off the pain of backache. It can also help you to relax and therefore loosen tense and aching muscles. For example, if you have difficulty getting to sleep at night take a portable cassette recorder into the bedroom and play music quietly. Specially recorded 'relaxation' music is available, but any kind of music that you like and find soothing will work just as well. It will distract you from thinking about the day's worries as well as your pain.

Why not take up an instrument yourself and play music instead of just listening to it. The piano and the guitar are two instruments which you can play for your own enjoyment, though it doesn't really matter what instrument you use as long as *you* find it relaxing.

POSTIVE THINKING AND ACTION

There are many different ways of coping with, and sometimes defeating, pain. The important thing to remember, as you will see from the case histories on pages 88 and 91, is to remain positive, never despair and to keep looking, with the assistance of your doctor, for new and alternative methods of pain control and relief. Never be worried that you are bothering your doctor too much, but enlist his or her support as you investigate new treatments.

Mary had suffered from backache ever since the birth of her second child. She had never been completely free from pain for eleven years. One doctor said she had damaged her ligaments. Another said she had muscle problems. No one could find any real explanation for her pain and, sadly, no one seemed able to offer her a permanent solution.

Early on, the doctor who had been caring for her at the time had prescribed a well-known tranquillizer for her; telling her that the pill was perfectly safe and would help to calm her and to reduce her pain. Like many doctors faced with a patient suffering from chronic, long-term pain Mary's doctor just did not know what to do. He thought that the tranquillizer would help a little because he recognized that Mary was anxious and a little depressed, and he knew that she was having difficulty in getting to sleep at night. Another (less justifiable) reason for the prescription was the fact that he really did not know what else to do for Mary. I am afraid that like most doctors he had never really been trained properly about how to help patients suffering from pain. (I don't mean to be rude about the medical profession, but there is no point at all in trying to hide the truth – particularly when many readers will know for themselves, and from their own experience, just how true this is.)

Mary, whose life had been made miserable by the pain, would have tried anything and was happy to take the tranquillizer – particularly since her doctor had convinced her that there would be no side effects.

Unfortunately, the drug the doctor prescribed was a benzodiazepine tranquillizer and within two months Mary was well and truly hooked!

Gradually, over the next two years she found that she needed to increase the dose of the tranquillizer. When she forgot to take one of the pills she suffered terrible withdrawal symptoms.

She found that whereas when she had first started to take the tranqillizers she had only been a little bit anxious and depressed, she became more anxious, more depressed and began to find it very difficult to get to sleep at night. If she missed a tablet by mistake she got a bad headache.

What Mary's doctor did not know was that the problems with the benzodiazepines had been identified some time ago, back in the early 1970s. It was discovered that these drugs produced all sorts of unpleasant and potentially dangerous side effects as well as being extremely addictive. Many experts had agreed that breaking the habit of taking benzodiazepine tranquillizers can be harder than getting off heroin or other illegal drugs.

Tragically, there is even evidence to show that the benzodiazepine tranquillizers are actually worse than useless for patients suffering from pain. In an experiment conducted by four research workers in the Behaviour Research Laboratory at Washington University it was even found that one of the most widely prescribed of all the many drugs in the benzodiazepine group could actually make some patients more sensitive to pain!

It took Mary nearly a year to wean herself off her tranquillizers. The doctor who had prescribed the drugs for her refused to help her. He told her that it was her own fault that she had become addicted.

After this experience Mary was reluctant to take drugs of any kind – but the backache still hadn't gone away and she desperately needed something to relieve her persistent pain.

So, she started to experiment with alternative pain control techniques.

She found, to her delight, even though she could not banish her pain completely (or, sadly, permanently) she could control it very effectively by using a mixture of techniques which she read about in a book dealing with 'natural' pain control techniques.

The technique she found most useful was a simple but effective one called 'visualization' (a technique which is described in this book under the heading *Use Your Imagination* on page 92). Another step forward was taken when Mary found herself a part-time, voluntary job working in a charity shop. Just keeping her mind busy seemed to make her less aware of her pain. The pain was still there, of course, but it didn't affect her life quite so much. Being busy kept up the sensory input to her brain, leaving less room for any pain sensations (I have described how this approach works under the heading *Keep Busy* on page 95).

THE BENEFITS OF MASSAGE

MASSAGE IS AN ANCIENT AND EXCELLENT WAY OF EASING TENSION, SOOTHING TIGHT MUSCLES AND RELIEVING PAIN. WHEN UNDER STRESS MOST PEOPLE FEEL THEIR MUSCLES TIGHTEN. THIS TENSION USUALLY AFFECTS THE MUSCLES IN THE NECK, SHOULDERS AND BACK. MASSAGE IS A VERY EFFECTIVE METHOD OF CLEARING AWAY MUSCLE 'KNOTS' AND RELIEVING MUSCLE STIFFNESS. MASSAGE ALSO HELPS TO STIMULATE THE PRODUCTION OF ENDORPHINS, THE BODY'S NATURAL PAIN KILLERS, AND STIMULATES THE PRODUCTION OF SENSORY IMPULSES WHICH THEN BLOCK THE TRANSMISSION OF PAIN MESSAGES. IN ADDITION, DOCTORS AND PSYCHOLOGISTS BELIEVE MASSAGE CAN SOOTHE THE MIND.

INSTRUCTIONS FOR A HOME MASSAGE

1. MAKE SURE YOU ARE COMFORTABLE. IF YOU ARE WEARING CLOTHES, THEY SHOULD BE LOOSE AND LIGHT.

2. KEEP THE ROOM TEMPERATURE PLEASANTLY WARM. IF THE TEMPERATURE IS TOO LOW YOUR MUSCLES WILL CONTRACT AND STIFFEN, AND THEY WILL BE DIFFICULT TO MASSAGE.

3. THE ROOM SHOULD NOT BE BRIGHTLY LIT.

4. SOME GENTLE BACKGROUND MUSIC MAY MAKE RELAXATION EASIER.

5. LIE DOWN ON THE FLOOR ON TOP OF A COUPLE OF RUGS. A BED OR SOFA WILL BE TOO SOFT AND SPRINGY TO MAKE THE MASSAGE EFFECTIVE.

6. IF YOU ARE GOING TO HAVE THE FRONT OF YOUR BODY MASSAGED PUT ONE PILLOW UNDER YOUR HEAD AND ANOTHER UNDER YOUR KNEES.

7. TO MAKE IT EASIER TO GIVE A MASSAGE, LUBRICATE THE SKIN WITH TALCUM POWDER OR OIL (ORDINARY BABY OIL WILL DO).

8. THE PERSON GIVING THE MASSAGE SHOULD START WITH A GENERAL MASSAGE. THEY SHOULD GENTLY STROKE AND KNEAD ALL YOUR MUSCLES; THEN THEY SHOULD CONCENTRATE ON SPECIFIC, PARTICULARLY TENSE PARTS OF YOUR BODY.

9. NEVER LET ANYONE MASSAGE YOUR JOINTS OR SPINE; THEY SHOULD STICK TO YOUR MUSCLES.

Cut Out Caffeine

Try to avoid drinking too much caffeine. It is probably the most widely used and most under estimated drug in the world today. The annual world-wide consumption of coffee – probably the commonest source of caffeine – is about 5 million tonnes. But caffeine is also an addictive and potentially dangerous stimulant which may increase your susceptibility to pain.

The Effects of Caffeine

1. It stimulates the brain and nervous system.

2. *It increases the effect of acid on the stomach.*

3. It makes the heart beat faster and raises the blood pressure.

4. *It opens up the lungs and it stimulates the kidneys.*

5. Too much caffeine can lead to muscle tremors, insomnia, anxiety, depression, headaches, indigestion, palpitations, bowel problems and personality changes.

Recommended Daily Intake

The daily intake for adults should not exceed 250 mg, and for children the daily intake should not exceed 125 mg.

- *A cup of ground coffee contains between 100 and 150 mg of caffeine.*

- *A cup of instant coffee contains between 75 and 100 mg of caffeine.*

- *A cup of tea contains between 50 and 100 mg.*

- *A mug of cocoa contains about 50 mg.*

- *Cola drinks can each contain 50 mg of caffeine.*

Like the vast majority of backache sufferers Simon has never found out the cause of his backache. But the pain ruled his life for seven years. He had to give up his work and all his hobbies. His sex life disappeared, and the constant pain gradually damaged his relationship with his wife so much that she eventually left him. Simon admits that his life had become totally ruled by his back problem. He could talk about little else.

Simon tried just about everything imaginable to control his pain. His doctor prescribed sixteen different

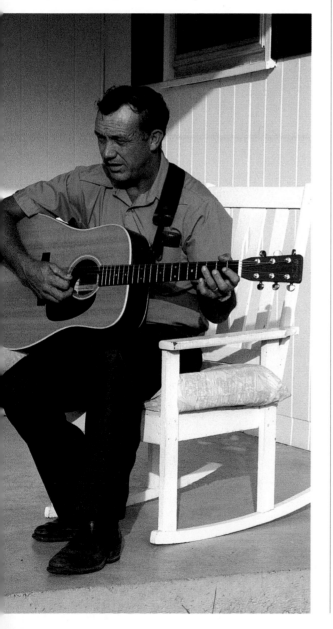

varieties of pain killer (I've seen his medical records and counted the prescriptions!). And Simon spent every spare penny he could raise on visits to acupuncturists, homoeopaths and herbalists. Sometimes he obtained a few days relief but nothing seemed to help very much in the long run.

Then Simon read about a pain clinic at a nearby hospital and persuaded his doctor to arrange for him to see a specialist there. Pain clinics are not really new but many patients who could benefit from them still haven't had the opportunity to do so.

The first pain clinics were developed by Dr John Bonica, an American doctor who was chief of anaesthesiology at a military hospital where the 7,700 beds were constantly full of soldiers who were suffering from war wounds. Every day the young doctor found himself struggling to find ways to help relieve the terrible pains of the men he was looking after. He talked to many other specialists at the hospital where he worked – gathering as much information as possible about the ways to conquer pain.

Today, most large hospitals have pain clinics where patients can be helped by doctors who usually have a considerable amount of specialist experience in the treatment of pain. Sadly, there are still not enough pain clinics – or enough pain specialists – but the medical profession has, at least, started to tackle pain in this professional way. I would recommend that any patient suffering from chronic pain ask his or her doctor to arrange a referral to the nearest pain clinic.

Simon benefited a tremendous amount from his visit to a pain clinic. The specialist he saw gave him a TENS machine to take home and try out and Simon found that he obtained more relief from this simple device than from any other pain control system. (I have described TENS machines on page 84).

ROCKING CHAIR

According to some experts one of the most effective ways to manage chronic low back pain is to sit in a rocking chair and 'rock around the clock'.

Using a rocking chair stimulates the production of nerve impulses which provide effective and continuous pain relief. Sitting in a rocking chair can be exremely soothing, restful and relaxing.

American President John F. Kennedy, who suffered from persistent backache, spent many hours sitting in the soothing comfort of a rocking chair when he was working in the White House.

KNOW YOUR ILLNESS

If you are worried about your pain or what is causing it then your anxiety will make your pain much worse than it need be.

Imagine, for example, that you have banged your head and acquired a headache. When you get home shortly afterwards you look in the mirror and notice that you have the beginnings of what will clearly end up being a fairly large bruise.

You may need to sit down and take things easy for a while. You may even take a couple of aspirin tablets; but you probably won't worry too much about the headache. You know what caused it and you know that it will almost certainly disappear fairly quickly.

Now, imagine that on your way home after banging your head you met a well-meaning friend who, when he hears that you have a headache, tells you that he once heard of someone who died of internal bleeding after a head injury similar to yours.

This time when you get home you won't be quite so calm about your headache. You'll begin to worry. You'll wonder about whether or not there could be any internal bleeding. Within an hour or so you'll be examining your limbs to see if there is any sign of developing weakness or paralysis.

Your anxieties will make your muscles so tense that your headache won't get better but will get worse. When you try to get to sleep you'll lie awake worrying. Eventually in desperation you'll pick up the telephone and call your doctor or you'll drag yourself down to the local hospital. There a doctor will examine your head, reassure you and tell you not worry.

Within minutes you will have relaxed, your tension will have evaporated and your headache will have gone!

A few years ago many doctors believed that patients were better off if they didn't know anything about their illness. But there is now a considerable amount of evidence to show that the truth is just the opposite: most patients suffer less pain and less anxiety if they are told what is wrong with them, what to expect and how best they can cope with their problems.

In one research project 97 patients who were in hospital for operations were all told exactly what to expect, exactly what sort of pain they would have to put up with and how best they would be able to combat that pain. After their operations these patients needed *half* the amount of painkilling medication required by another, similar group of patients who were given no information and no advice. The patients who were told what was happening to them were, on average, ready to go home a whole three days earlier than the other patients.

If you are in any doubt about what is causing your pain ask your doctor to tell you everything that he knows about your problem. If your doctor cannot give you the answers you want ask him to arrange for you to see a hospital specialist. If you still don't understand write down the name of the disease from which you are suffering and look up your problem in a book in your local library. It is perfectly natural to worry about your health if you are in pain, but the more you know about the cause of your pain and the more you understand what is going on, the less you will worry and the less pain you will suffer.

Remember that in many cases recurrent or persistent backache cannot be explained. Your doctors may not have been able to reach a diagnosis. But they will almost certainly have been able to exclude a number of potentially worrying disorders. And that information will probably be immensely reassuring. If you don't have to worry that you have something dangerous then you can concentrate on battling against your pain.

USE YOUR IMAGINATION

Until fairly recently most of the evidence linking the human imagination to pain was evidence showing that by thinking about sad and unhappy things, you could make yourself ill. However, you can actually use your imagination to help control your pain in a number of quite different ways.

First, you can use it to think of pleasant and relaxing scenes that help to calm and soothe you. You'll find more details about how to do this in Chapter Nine.

Second, you can use your imagination in a much more aggressive way. In one recent experiment patients were asked to concentrate on the parts of their bodies where their pains were most intense. They were then asked to visualize the shape of their pain and to imagine that it had a vivid red line all around it. The patients were then asked to watch their pain slowly getting smaller and smaller. The researchers found that as the patients imagined the pain area getting smaller, the intensity of their pain diminished.

By regarding your pain as an enemy, you can actually take a part in controlling it.

HERE ARE SOME PAIN CONTROL TECHNIQUES THAT HAVE BEEN SHOWN TO WORK

1. IMAGINE THAT YOUR MIND CAN DRIFT FREE OF YOUR BODY AND THAT YOU ARE ABLE TO WATCH YOURSELF FROM THE OTHER SIDE OF THE ROOM. YOU CAN SEE YOURSELF SURROUNDED BY CARING, COMPASSIONATE, GENTLE PEOPLE WHO ARE ALL DETERMINED TO HELP EASE YOUR PAIN. CONCENTRATE ON WHAT THEY ARE DOING AND ONLY RETURN TO YOUR BODY WHEN YOU SEE THAT THEY HAVE SUCCEEDED.

2. YOUR PAIN HAS BEEN TRANSFORMED INTO AN INVADING ARMY OF DIRTY BROWN CELLS. THE BETTER MENTAL PICTURE YOU HAVE OF THE 'ENEMY' CELLS THE MORE EFFECTIVE THIS TECHNIQUE WILL BE. IMAGINE THAT YOUR PAIN IS CAUSED BY THESE LITTLE SOLDIERS ATTACKING YOU WITH THEIR BAYONETS. NOW, IMAGINE THAT YOUR BODY'S OWN FIGHTING FORCES, YOUR WHITE CELLS, ARE REGROUPING TO ATTACK THE INVADERS. THEY HAVE BEEN QUIETLY BUILDING UP THEIR FORCES FOR SEVERAL HOURS AND ARE NOW READY TO TACKLE THE PAIN PRODUCERS. YOUR WHITE CELLS MARCH RESOLUTELY INTO BATTLE AND BEGIN TO DESTROY THE INVADING ARMY. IMAGINE THAT THE CORPSES OF THE BROWN CELLS ARE LITTERING YOUR TISSUES. YOUR WHITE CELLS MARCH THROUGH YOUR BODY IN TRIUMPH.

3. IMAGINE THAT DIFFERENT PARTS OF YOUR BODY ARE INSTRUCTED WHEN TO HURT BY A SERIES OF TELEPHONE CALLS FROM YOUR BRAIN. A NETWORK OF TELEPHONE WIRES CONNECT YOUR BRAIN TO EVERY SINGLE PART OF YOUR BODY THAT HURTS. BUT, DEEP INSIDE YOUR BODY A GROUP OF MINIATURE DOCTORS HAVE TAKEN OVER THE MAIN TELEPHONE EXCHANGE. EACH IS EQUIPPED WITH A PAIR OF WIRE CUTTERS AND THEY SYSTEMATICALLY SNIP THE WIRES TO CUT OFF THE CALLS. AS THE WIRES ARE CUT ONE BY ONE YOU REALIZE THAT YOUR PAIN IS BEING REDUCED.

IF YOU FIND ALL THESE TECHNIQUES DIFFICULT OR EVEN IMPOSSIBLE THEN YOU CAN BENEFIT ENORMOUSLY BY TAKING UP NEW HOBBIES OR INTERESTS THAT WILL PROVIDE YOU WITH A CHALLENGE. THE BUSIER YOU CAN KEEP YOUR MIND, THE MORE YOU CAN DO TO KEEP YOURSELF OCCUPIED, THE LESS YOU WILL NOTICE YOUR PAIN.

LEARN TO LAUGH

It may be an exaggeration to describe laughter as the best medicine. But it is no exaggeration to describe it as one of the best ways to tackle and defeat pain.

Scientists still don't know exactly how laughter does this but there are several theories. Some argue that laughter reduces the amount of inflammatory change in the human body. Others say that laughter helps by improving respiration, by lowering blood pressure and by increasing the supply of internally produced hormones. It may be that laughter works by just diverting attention away from pain.

Whatever the truth may be about how it works, there is little doubt that laughter – and even smiling – is an effective pain control therapy. And it has several advantages over other pain remedies: most notably it doesn't cost anything and there aren't any side effects.

Conquering pain through laughter doesn't just mean watching funny films and reading amusing books (though both those will help). You will find that you will benefit enormously if you can surround yourself with people who are generally happy and cheerful rather than sad and miserable. If you spend all your time with people who always look on the black side, who are always gloomy and pessimistic then you will inevitably begin to adopt their gloominess. Unhappiness is contagious.

And try not to take yourself – or everything in your life – too seriously. Of course, there will be some things in your life that you will want to take seriously, but that doesn't mean that you have to be serious all the time. It is good occasionally to watch a movie that has a message or to read a book that informs and educates. But it is also good to watch a movie that makes you laugh and to read a book that simply entertains. And remember that it isn't always the expensive things in life which provide the most pleasure. When did you last read a children's comic? When did you last stop and watch children playing about in the park? When did you last 'waste' an hour or two by the river?

If you are a naturally pessimistic individual try to suppress your pessimism and to replace it with at least a little optimism. Try to start each day in as cheerful a frame of mind as you can. If you get up in the morning

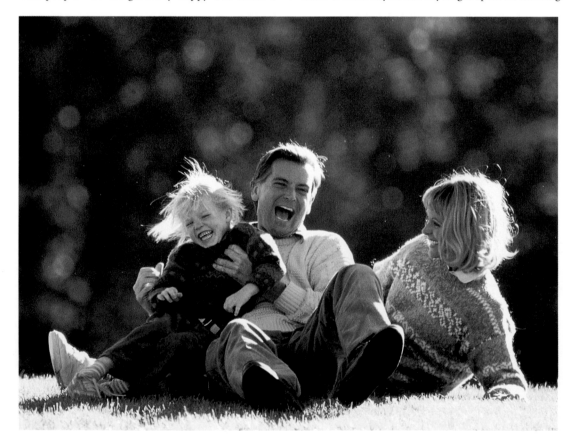

thinking of how your pain is going to restrict your life and how your backache is going to spoil everything you do, then it won't take much else to turn a potentially bad day into a terrible day. If you go through the day growling and scowling, then everyone you meet will be depressed by your mood and will respond accordingly. By evening you will be in a deep, dark depression. Your pessimism will have rebounded on you and rebuilt your fear, your misery and your susceptibility to pain. I know it isn't easy to be positive and for-ward-looking when backache has done a lot of damage to your life. But unless you are positive and optimistic backache will do even more damage.

"You will find that you will benefit enormously if you can surround yourself with people who are generally happy and cheerful rather than sad and miserable."

If you truly find it impossible to be optimistic or you find it difficult to smile or to laugh, then talk to your doctor and tell him how you feel. Depression and pain often go together in a vicious and debilitating cir-cle. Pain produces depression, and depression makes pain worse. It can be difficult to break the cycle but your doctor may be able to help you.

KEEP BUSY

Most people's natural reaction to pain is probably to rest. And when a pain is severe this is appropriate, sensible and healing.

Indeed, backache sufferers need to rest more than most pain victims since bedrest is often the only really effective way to deal with the problem.

But it is possible to rest too much. Unless your pain is acute or you have been told to rest by your doc-tor you may be doing yourself more harm than good by resting. Physical inactivity can result in the weakening of muscles and the deterioration of many of the body's essential organs, and can lead to the development of pressure sores. Mental inactivity can make pain worse simply by reducing the amount of sensory input going into your brain. If you have too little to think about then your brain will become ever more acutely aware of any pain sensations which might be around.

One of the earliest pieces of research to show the value of keeping your mind active was done by two researchers from the University of Oregon Medical School a few years ago. They took a number of volun-teer students and divided them into several groups. Members of the first group were told to sit still, to do nothing and to keep their hands in ice water for as long as they could. Members of the second group were also told to put their hands into ice water but were told that they could watch a nearby clock and use the clock to help set themselves goals and objectives. Members of the third group of volunteers were given access to a slide projector and a series of slides. They were allowed to operate the projector with their free hand and to look at as many slides as they liked.

The results of the experiment showed that when people in pain keep their minds busy they increase their pain tolerance level. The volunteers in the first group, the ones who were not thinking about anything in par-ticular, managed to keep their hands in the ice water for an average of 174 seconds. The volunteers in the second group, the ones who were watching the clock, managed to last out for 196 seconds. But the volunteers in the third group who were allowed to look at the slides managed to keep their hands in the ice water for an average of 271 seconds.

Clearly, therefore, you should do everything you can to keep yourself busy.

First, you should try to take as little time off work as possible. Work can provide you with physical activi-ty and mental stimulation as well as a target for your enthusiasm. The money can help too!

But if your work does not provide you with the intellectual stimulation that you need, then start taking evening classes or day classes at a local college. Try to find a subject that excites you and that you think you will enjoy. If it provides you with a useful skill as well then consider that a bonus.

When you need to distract yourself from your pain create mental games to keep your mind occupied if you don't have anything to read, watch or listen to. Try doing mental arithmetic or try concocting fantasies for yourself. It doesn't really matter what you do as long as you keep your mind busy.

WHAT IS PAIN?

Everyone knows what pain is but trying to produce a precise definition is a bit like trying to pick up a live fish in your bare hands. Just as you think you've got the thing under control it wriggles free, leaving you holding nothing. Pain is the single most important reason why people seek professional medical advice and the most common reason why they take pills. Yet it cannot be measured objectively.

Pain is neither a readily defined sensation nor a strictly regulated response. Between the original stimulus and the individual's perception of that stimulus a huge number of variables intervene – with the result that identical pain-producing stimuli can not only produce different responses in different individuals but can also produce different responses in the same individual on different occasions.

Your body's first response to a painful stimulus is to release a number of potent chemical substances. Normally stored in the body's tissues close to a comprehensive and sophisticated network of special nerve endings – which will eventually carry news about the painful stimulus to the brain and the rest of your body's nervous system – these chemicals stimulate those nerve endings almost immediately.

So, for example, if you are trying to hang a picture on a wall and you hit your thumb with a hammer the tissues of your thumb will immediately release two sets of chemicals known as kinins and prostaglandins. Both these substances sensitize your body's nerve endings and help ensure that messages are sent to your brain reporting the fact that your thumb has been hurt.

In addition to ensuring that these vital messages are transmitted as soon as possible the prostaglandins will also help increase the flow of blood to the part of your thumb that you hit. This sudden increase in circulation will result in your thumb turning red and starting to swell, and will bring white blood cells to the area to kill off any infective organisms which may have got in through a break in the skin. The swelling also results

in your thumb becoming difficult to move and therefore ensures that it will be rested while it recovers.

Whether you hit yourself with a hammer, stand on a nail or develop a boil, much the same sort of thing happens. In each case the inflammation or injury stimulates the local production of chemicals which ensure that your body's pain sensitive nerve endings carry the appropriate messages to your brain.

The pain receptors which are triggered by these chemicals and which pass the news on to your body's nervous system can be divided into several groups. There are receptors which carry information about extremes of heat or cold, and there are non-specific receptors which simply carry news of all ill-defined pains. There are even special receptors which detect the presence in your body of excess quantities of waste chemicals produced during hectic exercise.

Normally, these chemicals are removed by the circulating blood (that's one of the reasons why your heart rate goes up when you exercise), but if your circulation isn't powerful enough to remove the wastes as quickly as they are accumulating then special pain receptors will be stimulated.

Once your nerve endings have been triggered, the pain signal travels, partly as a chemical message and partly as an electrical impulse, along the appropriate nerve until it reaches the spinal cord. There the pain signal meets all sorts of other messages coming from other parts of your body and finally makes its way up your spinal cord to your brain.

The whole story of just how pain reaches your brain has long mystified scientists. The traditional theory, first made popular by Descartes in 1664, was that when a pain receptor is stimulated the pain message travels straight up to the brain. Descartes believed that it was all very simple – rather like a campanologist tugging on a bell rope to start the church bells ringing. This theory was popular with doctors until fairly recently, and many believed that in cases of intractable, long-term pain it would help to cut the nerves carrying the pain impulses up to the brain.

Unfortunately, this old-fashioned idea doesn't stand up very well. One major problem is that cutting the nerve doesn't stop pain impulses getting through and, indeed, may make the pain worse. A second problem is the fact that pain can continue long after the original stimulus has been removed. A third is that pain can occur spontaneously and may spread to apparently unrelated parts of the body. Finally, there is the problem that psychological factors can interfere quite dramatically with pain perception. Under some circumstances awful stimuli seem to produce no perceptible pain at all, whereas under other circumstances modest stimulations can produce really terrible pain. If we try to stick with the simple 'bell rope' theory of pain none of this seems to make any sense at all.

Then, in 1965 a psychologist called Ronald Melzack and an anatomist called Patrick Wall produced their 'gate control theory' which revolutionized the way doctors thought about pain.

Melzack and Wall claimed that only a certain amount of sensory information can be processed by the nervous system at any one time, and that when too much information tries to get through the limited number of junctions in the spinal cord means that some of the signals are shut out. The theory is that there is in the spinal cord a mechanism rather like a garden gate.

The gate control theory rests upon the fact that messages arrive at the spinal cord in three quite separate ways. First, there are the two main types of nerve fibre which detect pain and other sensations, and which carry electrical impulses produced by the receptors in the body's muscles and other tissues. The thicker of these two types of fibre carry sensations such as touch and pressure while the other thinner fibres carry pain messages. These two fibres differ in various ways: the thinner fibres can regrow if they are damaged, whereas the thicker fibres cannot regenerate and tend to diminish in number over the years. More importantly, the thicker fibres carry their nervous impulses much more rapidly than the thinner fibres do.

In addition to the messages travelling up towards your brain there are, of course, also likely to be instructions travelling down from the brain towards your muscles and other tissues.

"The 'gate control' theory helps to explain why pain is such an unpredictable force. And it shows why 'alternative' pain control techniques can be so effective."

Under normal circumstances the junctions or 'gates' in your spinal cord can carry these three different types of message quite comfortably, but if too many impulses reach the spinal cord at the same time the 'gates' just cannot cope: they shut down and won't accept any more messages at all.

It is this inability of the cells in the spinal cord to cope with the number of different messages they are getting which explains why some stimuli produce far more savage pains than other apparently comparable stimuli. It also explains how sometimes simply rubbing a sore or injured area can help get rid of the pain.

Imagine again that you have carelessly hit your thumb with a hammer. Your immediate reaction will be to rub the thumb vigorously. This means that there will now be two sorts of impulses racing along your nerves to try to get into your spinal cord and up to your brain: pain impulses, travelling along the thinner nerve fibres, and touch impulses, travelling along the thicker nerve fibres.

Inevitably, the 'gate' will be blocked and some impulses will be unable to get through. Since the touch impulses are travelling faster than the pain impulses they will get there first. Most of the pain impulses will be unable to get through.

There is another way in which the 'gate' can be become blocked.

If enough messages are coming down from the brain towards the tissues then the 'gate' will be blocked from the other side and, once again, the pain messages won't be able to get through. So, if you are concentrating very hard on what you are doing with your hammer you may not even notice that you've hit yourself until much later when you see the bruising! It is how a soldier can carry on fighting even though his foot has been shot off and how a man can pick up his severed arm and walk calmly with it to the nearest hospital. (Both true stories.) It also explains how two young lovers can stand outside in the freezing cold without noticing that they are getting frost-bitten!

Of course, if the number of impulses travelling along the smaller fibres carrying the pain messages greatly exceeds the number of fast-moving messages travelling along the larger fibres *and* the messages coming down from the brain, then the pain message will get through the 'gate', reach the brain, and you will become aware of the pain.

The 'gate control' theory helps to explain why pain is such an unpredictable and difficult force. And it also serves to show why 'alternative' pain control techniques can be so effective.

HIDDEN INFLUENCES – FACTORS WHICH AFFECT THE PAIN YOU FEEL

Have you ever come in from the garden, got into the bath and discovered that your arms and legs are covered in scratches and bruises? Have you ever been busy in the kitchen and then suddenly noticed that there is blood everywhere – from a finger you didn't even know you'd cut? In these instances pain impulses telling you to stop just couldn't get through the 'gate' because you were engrossed in what you were doing, and messages coming down from your brain telling your body what to do were blocking the pathways leaving no room for pain messages.

I have already described how pain impulses travel to your brain and can get held up, but there are other ways in which pain impulses can be hidden or arrested en route to your brain.

Most important is that for a pain to be felt the stimulus must exceed your personal pain threshold. If you are going to be aware that you have hit your thumb you must hit it with a certain amount of force. If you hit your thumb a light glancing blow, then you might be aware that your thumb has been 'touched' but you won't really feel a 'pain'. You do have to hit your thumb with a certain amount of force if your tissues are going to produce the chemicals necessary to stimulate a nervous response.

Pain thresholds vary from one individual to another. But, more important still, an individual's pain threshold varies from minute to minute according to a variety of hidden factors, some of which are described below.

WHETHER YOU ARE DEPRESSED

If you think a pain is trivial and harmless you will ignore it and it will probably go away. If you think a pain is serious and potentially life-threatening you will worry about it, and it will not go away. Your attitude towards the pain can be more important than the strength of the pain itself.

A patient called Mary who had undergone an operation for breast cancer five years earlier developed backache and was convinced that the cancer had reappeared and had invaded her spine. The pain was so bad that she could hardly move. But when X-rays showed that there was no sign of cancer – and no need to worry – Mary made an almost 'miraculous' recovery.

WHERE YOU ARE AND WHAT YOU ARE DOING

During a big football match not long ago one of the goalkeepers broke his neck, but he carried on playing! He was so wrapped up in the game that he ignored his pain until the match had finished. It was only then that he started to feel pain and he realized that he'd done something serious.

Your ability to tolerate pain goes up dramatically when you are busy doing something that holds your attention, and in one experiment volunteers found that they could put up with extra pain if they listened to music they liked.

HOW FRIGHTENED YOU ARE

Have you ever had a raging toothache, booked an appointment to see the dentist and found that by the time you walked into the consulting room your pain had completely disappeared?

You aren't alone if you have. It's very common.

When you are first aware of an aching tooth your threshold is low. You are worried by the pain and you don't know how long it is going to last or how severe it might become. Fear lowers your pain threshold and pain tolerance levels.

As soon as you've got your appointment to see the dentist your anxiety begins to lift. You feel more confident and because you know that relief will soon be available you suffer less from the pain.

YOUR ATTITUDE TOWARDS YOUR PAIN

Have you ever had a day when everything seems to go wrong? If you have then you know that by the end of it the smallest problem can become a crisis. A lost button, a missed bus or a mislaid pen can all seem horrendous. Small difficulties become out of all proportion when we feel low.

Your response to pain is influenced by your moods and emotions in exactly the same way. If you are feeling unhappy and you hit your thumb, then the pain will seem worse than if you are feeling happy when you hit your thumb.

YOUR SEX

Women have much the same sort of pain threshold as men but they are less tolerant of pain than men. This is probably because men are taught to be 'strong' and not to cry out when it pain.

On average men can tolerate pain for 20 per cent longer than women.

THE NUMBER OF BROTHERS AND SISTERS YOU HAVE

Children who grow up with at least three other brothers and sisters are likely to have much higher pain tolerance levels than children who grow up with fewer brothers and sisters.

Only children, on the other hand, are likely to grow up with lower pain threshold and pain tolerance levels than anyone else.

YOUR AGE

Your ability to tolerate pain will change as you get older. You will become better able to tolerate superficial pains and less able to tolerate deep pains.

WHAT YOU LEARNED AS A CHILD

Children are influenced by their parents.

If your parents made a fuss every time you got a bruise then you will have a comparatively low pain threshold and pain tolerance level. If, however, they took little notice when you complained of pain then you will have grown up indifferent to pain – with a high pain threshold and a great ability to tolerate pain.

Children can 'learn' pain behaviour from their parents. If you grew up in a household where one or both parents complained of back trouble you are more likely to suffer from back pain.

WHAT IS THE DIFFERENCE BETWEEN PAIN THRESHOLD AND PAIN TOLERANCE?

Your pain threshold level is the point at which you start to notice pain. Your pain tolerance level is the amount of pain you can stand.

PAIN IS USEFUL

You may find it difficult to believe – particularly if you've been kept awake all night by backache – but pain *is* useful.

Pain helps you to avoid serious injury. If you pick up a red hot pan you'll put it down quickly because it hurts. Without the pain you would have suffered a far more serious injury. Pain also helps to teach you which situations to avoid; when you've hit your thumb with a hammer you take more care.

Pain makes you rest parts of your body that might otherwise be damaged. If your knee hurts you'll rest it – and give it a chance to heal, and pain tells you when you need help. If you have persistent chest pain you see your doctor. If you have tooth pain you see the dentist.

PAIN THAT ISN'T WHAT IT SEEMS TO BE

If you close your eyes and someone sticks a pin in your thumb you will know where the pin is. You'll be able to locate the pin (and the pain) quite accurately.

Your ability to locate a pain, however, only works accurately when it is skin that has been injured. Pain that occurs inside your body can be very misleading.

If a disc 'slips' in your spine and presses on one of the nerves in your spinal cord that normally carries messages to and from your leg or foot, then you may think that you can feel pain coming from your leg or foot. There won't be anything wrong with your leg or foot, of course. The pain will be misleading and inappropriate. But the pain will be just as real as the pain you would get if you did injure your leg or foot.

CHAPTER SEVEN

Alternative Solutions

The popularity of alternative or complementary medicine has increased dramatically during the last few years, but patients wanting to try an alternative form of healing often have difficulty in getting answers to a few basic questions, such as: 'What sort of alternative medicine should I try?', 'Is it dangerous?' and 'Where do I find a good practitioner?'

The boom years of alternative medicine have seen the development of a huge number of strange and apparently 'new' specialities. Some of these specialities are, of course, well established. Acupuncture, for example, has been available for centuries and chiropractic dates from the end of the 19th century.

Others are much more modern and rely on the use of sophisticated-looking equipment. Some are variations on existing themes, and some are original. Some are designed to improve general health and others are designed to help treat specific problems.

"In any decent sized town you will find advertisements for acupuncturists and herbalists, osteopaths and homeopaths."

Some alternative specialities are based on unseen healing powers, while others rely on more traditional physical techniques using herbs or other drugs.

There has also been an explosion in the number of practitioners offering complementary health services. In any decent sized town you will find advertisements in local newspapers for acupuncturists and herbalists, osteopaths and homeopaths, chiropractors and hydrotherapists, reflexologists and hypnotherapists.

In many countries there are remarkably few laws about who can or cannot claim to be an 'alternative' medical practitioner.

Indeed, in huge areas of the world it is perfectly possible for someone with absolutely no qualifications to put up a brass plate on a Friday evening and to then open a 'clinic' on the following Monday morning after a weekend's study of a couple of books.

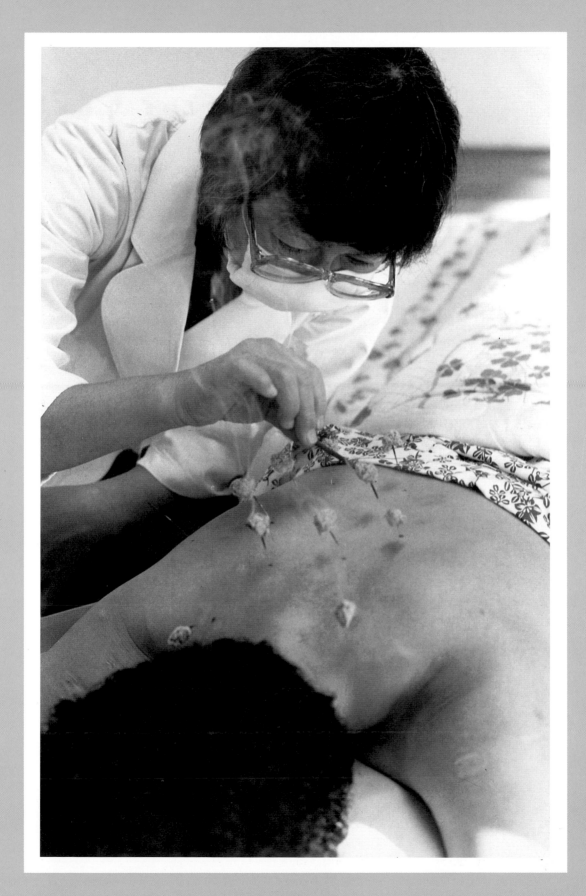

SOME BASIC RULES ON CONSULTING
AN ALTERNATIVE PRACTITIONER

1. IF YOU ARE UNSURE ABOUT WHAT IS WRONG WITH YOU THEN VISIT YOUR DOCTOR FIRST. ALTERNATIVE THERAPISTS ARE POOR AT MAKING DIAGNOSES AND CAN, ON OCCASIONS, MAKE VERY BASIC ERRORS. DOCTORS HAVE ACCESS TO DIAGNOSTIC EQUIPMENT – SUCH AS X-RAYS AND LABORATORY TESTS – THAT WILL PROBABLY BE UNAVAILABLE TO ALTERNATIVE PRACTITIONERS.

2. ALWAYS CALL YOUR DOCTOR IN AN EMERGENCY. ORTHODOX MEDICAL PRACTITIONERS ARE BY FAR THE BEST EQUIPPED TO DEAL WITH ACUTE CONDITIONS. AND IF YOU NEED TO GO INTO HOSPITAL YOU WILL HAVE TO SEE A DOCTOR.

3. ALTERNATIVE THERAPISTS ARE VERY GOOD AT DEALING WITH SPECIFIC PROBLEMS. FOR EXAMPLE, OSTEOPATHS ARE GOOD AT DEALING WITH BAD BACKS; ACUPUNCTURISTS WITH PERSISTENT AND APPARENTLY INTRACTABLE PAIN. HEALERS CAN HELP IMPROVE THE SURVIVAL CHANCES OF PATIENTS WHO ARE SUFFERING FROM LIFE-THREATENING DISORDERS. MASSAGE SPECIALISTS CAN HELP EASE MUSCLE ACHES AND PAINS. EXPERTS OFFERING RELAXATION TECHNIQUES CAN HELP PATIENTS CONQUER DISORDERS PRODUCED BY STRESS.

4. BY AND LARGE, ALTERNATIVE PRACTITIONERS ARE AT THEIR BEST WHEN DEALING WITH LONG-TERM MEDICAL PROBLEMS. THEY OFTEN GET THEIR BEST RESULTS WHEN FACED WITH PATIENTS WHO HAVE BEEN 'GIVEN UP' BY ORTHODOX DOCTORS.

5. BE SCEPTICAL WHEN SELECTING AN ALTERNATIVE PRACTITIONER. NEVER VISIT A PRACTITIONER WHO WORKS IN A BACK BEDROOM OR A LIVING ROOM, THEY SHOULD HAVE CLEAN AND PROPERLY EQUIPPED PREMISES. AND NEVER RELY ON ADVERTISEMENTS OR QUALIFICATIONS. THE BEST ORGANIZATIONS AND ASSOCIATIONS OF THERAPISTS OFTEN FROWN ON ADVERTISING BY THEIR MEMBERS. REMEMBER THAT THE PRACTITIONER WHO SEEMS TO HAVE A HOST OF EXCELLENT QUALIFICATIONS COULD WELL HAVE BOUGHT HIS IMPRESSIVE-SOUNDING DIPLOMAS OR UNDERGONE A BRIEF AND WOEFULLY INADEQUATE CORRESPONDENCE COURSE ON THE SUBJECT.

6. THE BEST WAY TO CHOOSE A GOOD LOCAL PRACTITIONER IS BY WORD OF MOUTH. ASK YOUR FRIENDS, RELATIVES AND NEIGHBOURS AND DON'T BE AFRAID TO ASK YOUR OWN FAMILY DOCTOR FOR ADVICE. RECENT RESEARCH HAS SHOWN THAT THE MAJORITY OF DOCTORS DO NOT DISAPPROVE OF THEIR PATIENTS SEEKING HELP FROM ALTERNATIVE THERAPISTS. YOUR OWN DOCTOR WILL PROBABLY KNOW WHICH LOCAL ALTERNATIVE THERAPISTS ARE RELIABLE AND HONEST, AND WILL BE ABLE TO STEER YOU AWAY FROM ANY WHO MAY BE INCOMPETENT AND UNSCRUPULOUS.

7. IN MY VIEW THERAPISTS IN THE FOLLOWING FIELDS CAN SOMETIMES OFFER USEFUL HELP FOR BACK PAIN SUFFERERS: ACUPUNCTURE, ALEXANDER TECHNIQUE, CHIROPRACTIC, HEALING, HOMOEOPATHY AND OSTEOPATHY.

ACUPUNCTURE

Acupuncture is one of the oldest established medical techniques in the world. It first started when ancient warriors began to notice that although they were being wounded by enemy arrows the pain of long standing aches and pains no longer gave them so much trouble. They gradually learned how and where to prick themselves with arrows to get rid of their chronic pains. Eventually thin bronze needles were invented to replace the arrows and today acupuncture needles are made of very thin stainless steel or copper.

Sadly, there are still many sceptics in the medical establishment who refuse to accept acupuncture because it is not a part of orthodox medicine. However, acupuncture treatment is widely available and the World Health Organization announced several years ago that it should be taken seriously

There is a considerable amount of evidence available now to show that acupuncture can, and often does, work. And backache (together with other bone and joint disorders) is one of the problems which is most likely to be treated effectively.

Although a massive amount of research has been done to try to find out how acupuncture works there is still a considerable mystery about this. The Chinese traditionally believe that the body has an internal energy force called 'chi' which flows around the body via a system of channels or meridians. Illness can be caused by one of the channels becoming blocked. They claim that acupuncture works by removing blockages through the insertion of needles into one or several of the 1000 acupuncture points around the body. This allows energy to travel more freely around the body. Other theories include those who believe that acupuncture may work by stimulating the patient's own body to produce endorphins - or natural, pain relieving hormones. A third group of scientists have suggested that acupuncture may work by blocking the pathways along which pain impulses are transmitted.

However acupuncture works there is no longer any doubt that it can, and frequently does, work.

It is, however, important to make sure that you visit a properly trained acupuncture specialist for in the wrong hands acupuncture needles can undoubtedly be dangerous. Before commencing treatment a skilled acupuncturist should ask you about your symptoms and make a diagnosis in much the same way as an orthodox doctor would.

There is, of course, the risk of contamination (there have been reported cases of patients in different parts of the world contracting both hepatitis and AIDS from dirty acupuncture needles) but that is by no means the only danger. Some highly trained experts in this speciality claim that acupuncture is such a powerful force that if used improperly or carelessly it can cause serious problems. However, if you choose your acupuncturist carefully the benefits far outweigh the dangers

HYDROTHERAPY

Many primitive societies believed in the curative powers of Holy Wells and springs. It is certainly true that both the Greeks and the Romans believed in the therapeutic value of bathing.

Today, after thousands of years, hydrotherapy is popular again and many backache sufferers swear by it.

After being out of fashion for many hundreds of years water therapy became fashionable in the eighteenth century when the practice of 'taking the waters' became a popular habit among the wealthy and among privileged members of society.

Today there are still a number of spa towns all over Europe which are treating patients for back ache and a wide range of other problems. In France, Germany, Italy and Britain there are a vast number of spa resorts where the weak and the ill can go to find succour, comfort and a hoped for cure.

Hydrotherapy comes in many different forms. The water can be used hot, cold or warm. It can be delivered by hose, by bucket or by drinking glass. It can be distilled and pure or quite rich in dissolved mineral salts. Patients can sit in baths, be massaged all over by underwater jets or take special showers. The type of treatment offered in establishments specializing in hydrotherapy is limited only by the imagination of the proprietor or doctor in charge.

Although very little proper clinical research has been done into the effectiveness of hydrotherapy there is no doubt that patients with joint troubles who are immobile out of water are often much more able to move in water where the effects of gravity are kept to a minimum. And, of course, warm water can be extremely relaxing to the muscles and the mind.

If you want to try hydrotherapy then you should be able to find a spa town or health farm with a heated swimming pool not too far away from you. And if you suffer from almost any type of joint, bone or muscle trouble then swimming around in warm, salty water will probably help you (though, as always, you should get your own doctor's approval first).

If your doctor approves then regular swimming in a warm pool should help keep your muscles toned..

If you don't want to visit a spa or health farm you should be able to find a local swimming pool which would be suitable. Or at the least you could try bathing in warm water at home. Try adding a few drops of aromatherapy oil for a really relaxing soak! Many thousands of people will confirm that resting in warm water will soothe the mind and ease aching muscles.

ALEXANDER TECHNIQUE

The Alexander Technique was founded at the turn of the century by an Australian actor called F. Matthias Alexander who believed that many common illnesses are caused by our failure to use our bodies properly.

Alexander started his researches when he repeatedly lost his voice on stage. Doctors were unable to help him and more and more often he found himself losing his voice in mid-performance.

Eventually, he realized that whenever he was talking he had developed a habit of stiffening his neck and pulling his head backwards and downwards. This meant that his vocal cords got squashed and when he tried to correct the problem by deliberately putting his head forwards he again found himself pressing on his vocal cords. After months off work Alexander decided that the only solution was to make an effort to change his posture and to hold his body in such a way that his voice could be saved.

The technique worked. Alexander found that once he had learned how to stand and how to hold his head his voice no longer kept on disappearing.

Alexander was so delighted by this discovery that he never returned to the stage. Instead he decided that since he had successfully managed to conquer his own problem by changing his posture, then there was a good chance that other people would also benefit by altering their posture. He created an educational programme aimed at eradicating bad posture and increasing self-awareness. The therapy (sometimes called the Alexander Technique and sometimes called the Alexander Principle) was designed to prevent illnesses developing, and to treat problems which had already developed simply by training individuals to use their bodies gracefully, sensibly and according to their natural, mechanical strengths and weaknesses. Teachers of the Alexander Technique are more interested in prevention than cure, and more adept at eradicating bad habits than in attacking existing symptoms directly.

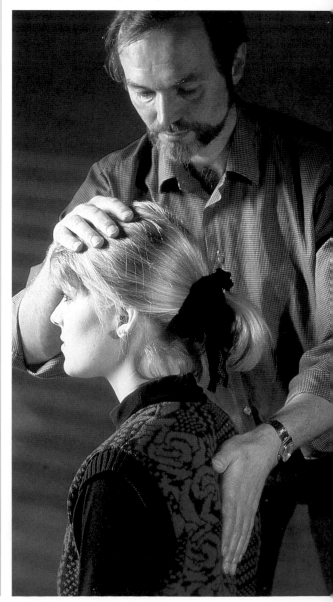

Like osteopathy and chiropractic the Alexander Technique is based on the belief that the position of the bones in particular, and the condition of the skeletal frame in general, can have a tremendous influence on the health of any individual.

Alexander believed that health can be restored and maintained simply by changing postural habits. He claimed that individuals who stand upright, with their backs straight and their heads held high, will have all their internal organs in exactly the right position. Such individuals would, he argued, be far less likely to develop any sort of disease or disorder. Alexander claimed that standing, walking and sitting properly would lead to a contented, comfortable and healthy lifestyle.

Today, teachers of the Alexander Technique still follow his theories closely. They help patients to use their natural reflexes to stand and move comfortably, and to use their bodies clearly, simply and effectively. The teachers assert that by improving posture and movement it is also possible to improve breathing, digestion and circulation.

The Alexander Technique is recommended for those suffering from a wide range of disorders, and patients with bone, joint and muscle disorders – particularly backache – are right at the top of the list of people most likely to benefit.

To get the best out of the Alexander Technique you need to visit a skilled and properly trained teacher. But it is possible to take advantage of some of Alexander's research without taking formal lessons.

Begin by trying to visualize the way that you stand, sit and walk. If you have a friend with a video camera then persuade him or her to take a few shots of you in various positions. These shots will enable you to assess your movements critically, objectively and clinically. Examine the sort of things you do in a normal day. Do you always move, lift and carry things without putting an unnecessary strain on your body? Do you sit, stand and walk properly? Look at your shoes to see if there is any sign of uneven wear. Remember that uncomfortable shoes or sore feet can affect the way that you walk and end up producing serious joint and spine problems. Remember not to over-reach when picking up heavy objects, and to lift heavy objects with your knees bent and your back straight.

CHIROPRACTIC

Chiropractic is the 20th-century equivalent of bone-setting, and it was established as a therapy in the last few years of the 19th century by a Canadian called Daniel David Palmer.

Palmer believed that 95 per cent of all illnesses were caused by displaced vertebrae (the technical term he used for displacement was 'subluxation'), and after managing to restore the hearing of a janitor who had been deaf for 17 years, Palmer was convinced that the spine was the key to good health and that spinal manipulations would deal with most if not all illnesses.

However, because of Palmer's rather extreme views chiropractic was, from the start, generally opposed by the medical establishment.

Today chiropractors still believe that when parts of the body's bony frame are displaced they can press against nerves – causing pain and many other symptoms. Some chiropractors claim that by manipulating bones and joints they can not only help deal with specific structural problems but also help relieve internal problems involving non-bony organs, such as the heart and lungs, although many chiropractors admit that chiropractic cannot deal with all ailments and is best suited for the treatment of disorders of the bones and joints – particularly backache, neck, shoulder and arm pains and headache.

Traditionally chiropractors use their hands to help them reach a diagnosis, but many modern chiropractors also use X-rays to help decide exactly what is wrong with their patients.

Treatment from a chiropractor usually involves manipulation, and since manipulation of the spine can be dangerous if done carelessly or if it is not preceded by the proper investigations, it is very important to make sure that the chiropractor you see knows what he or she is doing.

HEALING

'Miraculous cures rejected by doctor', said the headlines recently when a doctor was reported to have announced that although he had spent 20 years examining the phenomenon of healing, he had not found a single case comparable to the miracles of Christ.

I was sad but not surprised, and would respectfully

suggest that maybe the good doctor hasn't been looking hard enough. Maybe he's too much in awe of good old-fashioned 'if-you-can't-explain-it-then-it-doesn't-exist' science to accept that the word 'impossible' is really little more than a synonym for 'inexplicable'.

Maybe, too, the doctor has too much awe for the miracles of Christ. Would they, I wonder, stand up to rigorous examination under the eyes of the professionally qualified sceptic? Where are the clinical notes that prove that the man who picked up his bed really was paralysed and wasn't suffering from viral encephalitis or some psychosomatic disorder?

I'm not being deliberately provocative but I have to confess that to me it doesn't seem wise to talk about the miracles of Christ as though they were beyond all scientific doubt.

The medical profession and the church have much in common. They both like secrecy and abhor competition of any kind. They both demand evidence from others that they themselves can rarely provide. They both have a fear and dislike of things which are outside their control. Those who dismiss healing as an unlikely phenomenon will find many supporters among the medical and clerical establishments.

I'm afraid, however, I have far more faith in miracles than I have in many doctors or spokesmen for the church. Maybe that's because before I became a professional author I worked as a general practitioner and saw far too many things that medicine could not explain.

The medical profession may not like the idea that people can be healed without pills, and the church may find all the competition a bit unnerving, but the plain fact is that things which doctors and scientists cannot explain do happen quite regularly.

How else would you describe what happened to Pam? She had cancer of the bowel and should have died within a matter of weeks according to the hospital specialists who were helping to look after her. But she didn't die. She wasn't married but she did have three small children to take care of, and she wasn't ready to die. So while the doctors did more and more laboratory

"Those who dismiss healing as an unlikely phenomenon will find many supporters among the medical and clerical establishments."

tests which showed that she should have been dead she just carried on looking after her family.

I can tell you lots of true stories like that as, I'm sure, can thousands of other general practitioners.

No one in the medical profession took the credit for Pam's miraculous recovery. She and her God simply did whatever needed to be done between them.

But I've seen miracles with my own eyes that have been claimed by healers and I believe them, too.

What little scepticism I had disappeared a few years ago when I was making a series of TV programmes. Just before starting the series I received a letter from a lady who claimed to be a healer. I invited her into the studios and she brought with her a patient who had suffered from bad arthritis and who claimed that her pains had miraculously disappeared.

Clinically the evidence was very impressive. The patient appeared to be in perfect health, but it was the X-ray evidence that I found the most convincing.

I'd managed to obtain the patient's X-rays from her hospital consultant and they proved that her arthritis had been inexplicably but undeniably healed. I also consulted an expert radiologist who agreed with me that there had been a definite change in the patient's X-rays after she had seen the healer.

I've seen 'miracles' work the other way too.

How, I wonder, would the sceptics explain the perfectly healthy patient who, after being mistakenly told that he had incurable cancer, started to die? And how would sceptics explain the fact that when the man was told of the mistake he quickly got better again?

If you don't like the idea of the unknown I can offer you explanations for these apparent miracles.

Scientists have known for years that the human body contains a massive range of self-healing mechanisms – including its own supply of a morphine-like painkiller – so it seems logical that healers are simply people who have found a way to stimulate the body's own self-healing mechanisms.

Those sceptics who say that healing is in fact all in

the mind – and only works because people want it to work – must also somehow explain the research which has shown that healers can also help animals and even plants get better quicker.

Most doctors readily accept that people can make themselves ill by worrying, and no doctor worth his salt would deny the efficacy of the placebo effect – where patients get better when given sugar pills. Some scientists have even gone a long way towards proving that miracles do happen.

Dolores Krieger, now a doctor but at the time a Professor of Nursing at New York University, has convinced many sceptical doctors by running controlled clinical trials in which blood pressure changes produced by a 'laying on of hands' are measured in a laboratory.

Ten years ago doctors would have scoffed at the idea that patients could be 'healed'. Today a growing number of doctors – both hospital doctors and general practitioners – are using 'healers' and 'healing' as commonly as they use drugs and surgery.

Indeed, in an attempt to prove to the few remaining sceptics that healing really does work, a number of research projects are currently taking place in British hospitals – designed to show exactly how effective healing can be.

No one pretends to understand how healing works, but it is one of the fastest-growing medical specialities. And very few doctors are now prepared to deny that it does work.

There are at least 7000 healers working in Britain today. Just to put things in perspective, that is more than the number of surgeons working in British hospitals.

The truth is that by telling the world that miracles don't happen there is a danger that patients will lose the hope that they are entitled to. And because miracles happen best (though not exclusively) when people believe that there is still hope for them, those who dismiss modern miracles are, in my view, doing far more harm than good.

Of course, sometimes the enthusiastic supporters of healing do get a bit carried away, and some of the claims that are made are probably over the top. But none of this is new. Clovis the Frank was holding special healing sessions in A.D. 496, and the 11th-century Anglo-Saxon king Edward the Confessor had his subjects queuing for days in the hope that a touch from a royal finger would cure them.

Many healers are so thrilled by their powers and their successes in curing the sick that they work free of charge. 'Healing,' one healer told me, 'is not a special gift. It's just that full-time healers practise a lot and get quite good at it. We don't think it is something we should charge money for.'

Do you think you might have the healing touch? Here is a way to find out.

With your arms at right angles to your body you should place your hands very close together, palms facing eachother but not quite touching. Your fingers should point away from your body.

Now move your hands a few inches in opposite directions and hold them apart for a few seconds. Then return them to the starting position – very close together but not touching. Maintain this position for a few seconds and then separate them by a few inches more than the first time. Once again keep them apart for a few seconds.

After returning your hands to the original position separate them by six inches. Do this as slowly as you can.

Finally, separate your hands by eight or ten inches and gradually bring them back together again in a series of jerky, two-inch movements.

Do you feel a strange bounciness? If you have the healing touch you will notice that your hands either become warmer or cooler, or start to tingle.

To use your own healing powers simply place your hands on or close to your patient's body. And then simply project a feeling of well-being, comfort, happiness, good will and good health from your body to theirs.

Do remember though that healing isn't an alternative to orthodox medicine. It's an 'extra' – something done to help and not replace the doctors who are looking after your patient.

" A growing number of doctors - both hospital doctors and general practitioners - are using 'healers' and 'healing' as commonly as they use drugs and surgery."

HOMOEOPATHY

The principles of homoeopathy go back to the origins of medicine, but the principles of modern homoeopathic practice were established by Samuel Hahnemann in the early part of the 19th century.

It was known then that cinchona bark (which contains the drug we now know as quinine) relieves the symptoms of the ague (a disorder now known as malaria). Even though he did not have the ague Hahnemann decided to see what would happen when he took some quinine himself. He was startled to discover that when he took the drug he developed the fever and the other symptoms normally associated with the disease. In due course he noticed that the symptoms of the disease disappeared when he stopped taking the drug.

Hahnemann knew that according to Hippocrates if an individual who is suffering from an illness can be made to suffer symptoms similar to those produced by his illness then he will be cured. This is the ancient theory of 'like curing like', also known as the law of similars. Hahnemann realized that quinine satisfied this law and immediately set about trying to find more drugs that had a similar effect.

"In homeopathy the treatment is designed to fit the patient, not the disease."

Over 2000 years ago Hippocrates wrote that 'through the like, disease is produced, and through the application of the like it is cured.' Paracelsus, who was a vital figure in the re-emergence of medicine as a science during the Renaissance, said much the same thing. Hahnemann's basic principle is that 'a substance which produces symptoms in a healthy person cures those symptoms in a sick person'. During the following few years he experimented with all sorts of things: metals, salts, animal products and vegetable substances. He discovered an enormous range of products which fitted his theory and which could be used to produce symptoms similar to those associated with specific disorders.

As he continued his research Hahnemann also discovered that he did not need to use large doses of his medicines in order to obtain the desired effects. Indeed, on the contrary, to his great surprise he discovered that the smaller the dose he used the more effective it was. And thus homoeopathy was born.

Today the theory behind homoeopathy remains exactly the same. Minute doses of drugs are given with the intention of triggering off some sort of defensive reaction within the body and of stimulating the body's natural resistance to disease. Homoeopathy has, it seems, a good deal in common with vaccination, in which a small amount of an infective organism is introduced into the patient's body in order to stimulate the body's own defence mechanisms to prepare suitable defences against disease.

The dilutions that homoeopathic practitioners use for treatment are so small that in order to prepare their medicines homoeopathic practitioners effectively empty a bottle of concentrated medicine into a lake and then use the lake water as medicine.

For a homoeopath, making the correct diagnosis is a vitally important starting point. The first interview you have with a homoeopath is likely to take as long as two hours. The questions a homoeopath will ask will cover a wide range of mental, physical and emotional issues, for the homoeopath aims to find out as much as he possibly can about his patient as an individual. It is only by this sort of lengthy and exhaustive questioning that the homoeopath can decide what sort of treatment to use because in homoeopathy the treatment is designed to fit the patient, not the disease.

The medicine that is chosen must be one that will suit the patient's psychological make-up, temperament and lifestyle. The homoeopath will be keen to find out what changes you have experienced in recent weeks. He will want to know about your personal feelings and any behavioural changes that you – or your friends or relatives – have noticed. He will have to know about your needs and fears if he is to choose the correct treatment. The homoeopath will want to know also how you respond to the temperature, the weather, the environment and the time of the day.

Homoeopaths believe that symptoms are a sign that the body is fighting a danger of some kind, and to provide the correct treatment the homoeopath needs to know as much as possible about your strengths and weaknesses so that he can give the right sort of help.

In order to evaluate new possible treatments homoeopaths have to do 'provings' of potentially useful substances. To do this they give very small doses of animal, vegetable or mineral substances to healthy people for several weeks (in just the same sort of way that Hahnemann tried out quinine on himself). During that time the experimenters will need to record any symptoms which are produced.

By the time he died in 1843 Hahnemann had done 'provings' on 99 different substances. By the year 1900 over 600 more medicines had been added to the list of useful remedies. And today there are around 3000 substances available to homoeopaths. The diversity of materials used includes onions, Indian hemp, gold, copper, mercury, sulphur, cadmium, honey-bee-sting venom, snake venom and spiders.

Once the homoeopath has made his diagnosis then he must choose the correct substance from this list of possible remedies. Usually homoeopaths prefer to use a single cure, however many symptoms you may have. If you go to see a homoeopath complaining of a headache and diarrhoea, as well as a backache, then the homoeopath will try to give you one remedy to treat all three problems rather than three separate remedies. The homoeopath always has to remember that it is the patient – not the disease – that he is treating.

There are many mysteries about homoeopathy. How does it really work? How are such diluted medicines able to have any useful effect on the human body? How is it that the more diluted a homoeopathic medicine is the more powerful it seems to be?

There are no answers to these questions. But there is now evidence available to prove that homoeopathy really does work.

One of the main reasons why Samuel Hahnemann was keen to develop homoeopathy was that he was disenchanted with the medicines available to his medical colleagues at the start of the 19th century. Hahnemann knew only too well that patients treated by orthodox means were often made worse by being given huge doses of potentially harmful drugs. He wanted to find a technique that would reduce the risk of patients developing unpleasant or dangerous side effects.

It is this high level of safety – and scarcity of side effects – which today makes homoeopathy so popular among patients and among health care professionals. If you want to try this form of treatment you should have no difficulty in finding a properly trained practitioner.

OSTEOPATHY

Some osteopaths trace their profession back hundreds of years from the simple, roving surgeons of early times and through the bone-setters of the 18th century. It was not, however, until the year 1874 that the founder of modern osteopathy, Andrew Taylor Still, made public his theories.

Still was an American, the son of a Methodist preacher, and he hated drugs and alcohol of all kinds. He firmly believed that the human body can be treated as a machine and that faults in the musculo-skeletal system are responsible for the development of a huge variety of diseases. Although one of Still's early students, a man called John Martin Littlejohn, tried to expand the basis upon which osteopathy was founded, most of Still's followers believed that they could help their patients best by manipulating their spines.

Today, although a small number of osteopaths will claim that they can help alleviate a wide range of problems, the majority of practising osteopaths concentrate simply on dealing with backache, leg pains, headaches and neck pains by manipulating bones and joints. Over half of all the patients who visit osteopaths have one particular problem: backache.

Osteopaths diagnose their patients by watching the way that they walk, stand and sit; by taking a full personal history; by performing a physical examination; and by taking X-rays. Treatment is usually done with massage and manipulation. Osteopaths stretch and move their patients' joints in all directions.

Osteopathy isn't completely safe. The manipulation of joints can lead to problems. To reduce the risk osteopathy needs to be carried out with great care. It should only be used after a thorough diagnosis has ruled out the possibilities of there being some condition (such as a fracture, a tumour or an infection) which makes manipulation unwise.

Osteopathy is an excellent form of treatment for simple bone, joint and muscle problems. Most doctors with backache visit osteopaths or chiropractors for treatment themselves.

CHAPTER EIGHT

The Importance Of Relaxation

Stress, tension, anxiety, worry and pressure are among the most common causes of backache. Millions of men and women who suffer constantly from back pain do so not because of any bony injury nor because their joints are unduly worn, but because the muscles of their backs are tired, strained and in spasm. Amazingly, as many as eight out of ten cases of backache are caused by the tensions of stress!

Whenever you are worried or under stress your body responds in much the same way: your heart beats faster, your blood pressure goes up and your muscles become tight and tense.

"Whenever you are worried or under stress your body responds in much the same way: your heart beats faster, your blood pressure goes up and your muscles become tight and tense."

Your body reacts in this simple and fairly primitive way because the only sort of stress it is designed to respond to is a physical one. When your body recognizes that your mind is worried it assumes that you are facing a real, physical danger and it prepares itself accordingly to respond to this danger.

Your heart rate and blood pressure go up so that you will be better able to fight for your life – or to run away from a predator. At the same time acid pours into your stomach to turn any food there into energy, and your muscles become tense and tight so that you will be perfectly equipped to fight your enemy or run away.

Sadly, however, most modern threats are not physical ones and you cannot run away from redundancy or a failed marriage or fight a gas bill. Your physical response to such stresses is quite inappropriate. But your body doesn't know that, and it continues to respond in a real, physical way for as long as the threat continues.

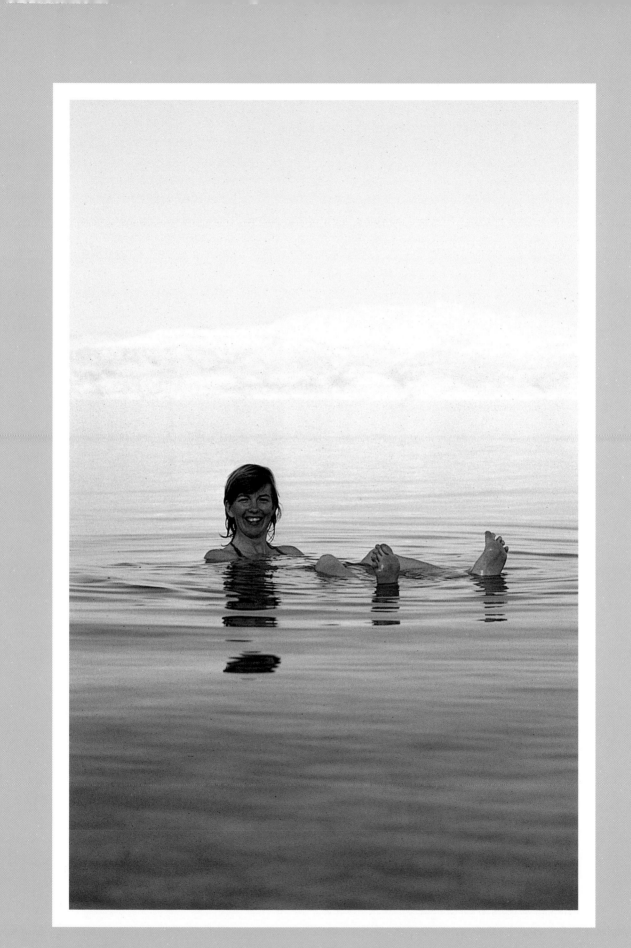

So, if you get stuck in a traffic jam your muscles will remain tense for hours. If you have a higher pressure job (or no job at all) or you are constantly worried about money your muscles will stay tense and tight for hours, days, weeks and months on end.

The symptoms you get will depend on the part of your body which suffers first. If it is the muscles around your head which are constantly tensed then you will get a headache. If it is the muscles around your bowels which suffer most then you will probably suffer from the irritable bowel syndrome. But if it is the muscles of your back which respond most dramatically to the stresses in your life, you will suffer from backache. If you have a job which involves a lot of sitting down, a lot of driving or travelling or a lot of bending over the sink or the cooker, then your back muscles will be under an extra strain, and the chances of their suffering first will be increased enormously.

You can deal with the sort of stress and pressure that tightens up your back muscles in two ways: by learning how to relax your muscles directly or by learning how to relax your mind (and thereby relaxing your muscles indirectly).

How To Relax Your Body

Learning how to avoid unnecessary stresses and tensions, build up your resistance to stress and improve your ability to cope with stress will all help you in your fight against muscle tension.

But there is another more direct way to tackle muscle tension and the associated problems it produces: deliberately relaxing your tensed muscles.

If you decide to try to learn how to relax your body please do not make the mistake of assuming you can learn how to do it usefully and effectively just by reading through these lines once.

Learning how to relax requires some effort and concentration and so you will need to practise this technique several times before you really begin to benefit from it. You should, however, learn how to relax yourself physically in no longer than it takes to learn how to dance, swim, play tennis or drive a car.

And once you have learned how to relax you will have acquired a valuable skill which will stay with you for life and will benefit you enormously.

Relaxing Your Body

MAKE SURE THAT YOU WILL NOT BE DISTURBED FOR AT LEAST 20 MINUTES, THEN LIE DOWN SOMEWHERE QUIET AND COMFORTABLE, AND USE THIS SIMPLE-TO-LEARN TECHNIQUE TO HELP RELIEVE MUSCLE TENSION.

1. TAKE VERY DEEP, SLOW BREATHS. STRESS WILL MAKE YOU BREATHE MORE QUICKLY THAN USUAL SO SOOTHE YOUR MIND – AND YOUR BODY – BY DELIBERATELY TAKING SLOWER, DEEPER BREATHS.

2. CLENCH YOUR LEFT HAND AS TIGHTLY AS YOU CAN, MAKING A FIST WITH YOUR FINGERS. DO IT WELL AND YOU WILL SEE THE KNUCKLES GO WHITE. IF YOU NOW LET YOUR FIST UNFOLD YOU WILL FEEL THE MUSCLES RELAX. WHEN YOUR HAND WAS CLENCHED THE MUSCLES WERE TENSED; UNFOLDED THE SAME MUSCLES ARE RELAXED. THIS IS WHAT YOU MUST DO WITH THE OTHER MUSCLE GROUPS OF YOUR BODY.

3. BEND YOUR LEFT ARM AND TRY TO MAKE YOUR LEFT BICEPS MUSCLE STAND OUT AS MUCH AS YOU CAN. THEN RELAX IT AND LET THE MUSCLES EASE. WHEN YOUR ARM IS THOROUGHLY RELAXED LET IT LIE LOOSELY BY YOUR SIDE.

4. CLENCH YOUR RIGHT HAND AS TIGHTLY AS YOU CAN, MAKING A FIST AGAIN WITH YOUR FINGERS. WHEN YOU LET YOUR FIST UNFOLD YOU WILL FEEL THE MUSCLES RELAX.

5. NOW BEND YOUR RIGHT ARM AND MAKE YOUR RIGHT BICEPS MUSCLE STAND OUT AS MUCH AS YOU CAN. THEN RELAX IT AND LET THE MUSCLES BECOME RELAXED. WHEN YOUR ARM IS THOROUGHLY RELAXED LET IT LIE LOOSELY BY YOUR SIDE.

6. TIGHTEN THE MUSCLES IN YOUR LEFT FOOT. CURL YOUR TOES UPWARDS. AND THEN DOWNWARDS. WHEN YOUR FOOT FEELS AS TENSE AS YOU CAN MAKE IT DELIBERATELY RELAX THE MUSCLES.

7. TENSE THE MUSCLES OF YOUR LEFT CALF. YOU SHOULD BE ABLE TO FEEL THE MUSCLES IN THE BACK OF YOUR LEFT LEG BECOME FIRM AND HARD . BEND YOUR FOOT UP TOWARDS YOU TO HELP TIGHTEN THE MUSCLES. THEN LET THE MUSCLES RELAX.

8. STRAIGHTEN YOUR LEFT LEG AND POINT YOUR FOOT AWAY FROM YOU. YOU WILL FEEL THE MUSCLES ON THE FRONT OF YOUR LEFT THIGH TIGHTEN UP – THEY SHOULD BE FIRM RIGHT UP TO THE TOP OF YOUR LEG. NOW RELAX THOSE MUSCLES AND LET YOUR LEFT LEG LIE LOOSELY ON THE BED.

9. TIGHTEN THE MUSCLES IN YOUR RIGHT FOOT. CURL YOUR TOES UPWARDS. AND THEN DOWNWARDS. WHEN YOUR FOOT FEELS AS TENSE AS YOU CAN MAKE IT DELIBERATELY RELAX THE MUSCLES.

10. TENSE THE MUSCLES OF YOUR RIGHT CALF. YOU SHOULD BE ABLE TO FEEL THE MUSCLES IN THE BACK OF YOUR RIGHT LEG BECOME FIRM AND HARD AS YOU TENSE THEM. BEND YOUR FOOT UP TOWARDS YOU TO HELP TIGHTEN THE MUSCLES. THEN LET THE MUSCLES RELAX.

11. STRAIGHTEN YOUR RIGHT LEG AND POINT YOUR FOOT AWAY FROM YOU. YOU WILL FEEL THE MUSCLES ON THE FRONT OF YOUR RIGHT THIGH TIGHTEN UP – THEY SHOULD BE FIRM RIGHT UP TO THE TOP OF YOUR LEG. NOW RELAX THOSE MUSCLES AND LET YOUR RIGHT LEG LIE LOOSELY ON THE BED.

12. LIFT YOURSELF UP BY TIGHTENING YOUR BUTTOCK MUSCLES. YOU SHOULD BE ABLE TO LIFT YOUR BODY UPWARDS BY AN INCH OR SO. THEN LET YOUR MUSCLES FALL LOOSE AGAIN.

13. TENSE AND CONTRACT YOUR ABDOMINAL MUSCLES. TRY TO PULL YOUR ABDOMINAL WALL AS FAR IN AS POSSIBLE, THEN LET GO AND ALLOW YOUR WAIST TO REACH ITS MAXIMUM CIRCUMFERENCE.

14. TIGHTEN UP THE MUSCLES OF YOUR CHEST. TAKE A BIG, DEEP BREATH IN AND STRAIN TO HOLD IT FOR AS LONG AS POSSIBLE. THEN, SLOWLY, LET IT GO.

15. PUSH YOUR SHOULDERS BACKWARDS AS FAR AS THEY WILL GO, THEN BRING THEM FORWARDS AND INWARDS. FINALLY, SHRUG THEM AS HIGH AS YOU CAN. KEEP YOUR HEAD PERFECTLY STILL AND TRY TO TOUCH YOUR EARS WITH YOUR SHOULDERS. IT WILL PROBABLY BE IMPOSSIBLE BUT TRY ANYWAY. THEN LET YOUR SHOULDERS RELAX AND EASE.

16. NEXT TIGHTEN UP THE MUSCLES OF YOUR BACK. TRY TO MAKE YOURSELF AS TALL AS YOU CAN. THEN LET THE MUSCLES RELAX.

17. THE MUSCLES OF YOUR NECK ARE NEXT. LIFT YOUR HEAD FORWARDS AND PULL AT THE MUSCLES AT THE BACK OF YOUR NECK. TURN YOUR HEAD FIRST ONE WAY AND THEN THE OTHER. PUSH YOUR HEAD BACKWARDS WITH AS MUCH FORCE AS YOU CAN. THEN LET THE MUSCLES OF YOUR NECK RELAX. MOVE YOUR HEAD AROUND AND MAKE SURE THAT YOUR NECK MUSCLES ARE COMPLETELY LOOSE.

18. MOVE YOUR EYEBROWS UPWARDS AND THEN DOWN AS FAR AS THEY WILL GO. DO THIS SEVERAL TIMES, MAKING SURE THAT YOU CAN FEEL THE MUSCLES TIGHTENING. THEN RELAX.

19. SCREW UP YOUR EYES AS TIGHTLY AS YOU CAN. PRETEND THAT SOMEONE IS TRYING TO FORCE YOUR EYES OPEN. KEEP THEM SHUT TIGHTLY. THEN, KEEPING YOUR EYELIDS CLOSED, LET THEM RELAX.

20. MOVE YOUR LOWER JAW AROUND. GRIT YOUR TEETH. WRINKLE YOUR NOSE. SMILE AS WIDE AS YOU CAN SHOWING AS MANY TEETH AS YOU CAN. PUSH YOUR TONGUE OUT AS FAR AS IT WILL GO, PUSH IT FIRMLY AGAINST THE BOTTOM OF YOUR MOUTH AND THEN THE TOP OF YOUR MOUTH BEFORE LETTING IT LIE EASY AND RELAXED INSIDE YOUR MOUTH. NOW LET ALL YOUR FACIAL MUSCLES GO LOOSE AND RELAXED.

MAKE YOUR OWN RELAXATION TAPE

To make your own relaxation tape slowly read out the 'Relaxing Your Body' script into a tape recorder. Then lie down, play back the tape and listen to it carefully. You'll find it much easier to listen to the instructions on a tape than to try and read them out of a book while you are relaxing. Do remember to read out the instructions fairly slowly – and to pause between each set of instructions. You may need one or two attempts to get it absolutely right.

WARNING
WHEN YOU HAVE RECORDED YOUR TAPE DO **NOT** LISTEN TO IT WHILE DRIVING OR OPERATING MACHINERY SINCE IT MAY MAKE YOU DROWSY.

HOW TO RELAX YOUR MIND

There is no doubt that stress causes many people to suffer backache. However, more often than not, the imagination used in a negative and destructive manner creates a level of stress that is totally out of proportion to the problems most people face in life.

The mind is incredibly powerful and people are easily led astray from reality by the power of suggestion. For example, you may get stressed about something that should be enjoyable, like throwing a party. At first, it seems like a good idea, then as the day approaches you begin to feel a little nervous. Have you got the right mix of people? What are you going to wear? How much is it going to cost? When the day arrives, you may begin to worry about the amount of food you have prepared and who is actually going to turn up. A couple of guests phone to say they cannot make it. All of a sudden you grow tense. Your imagination runs wild and it occurs to you that, in the worst case, no one is actually going to turn up at all. By the time the first guests ring the doorbell, you are in a real panic and probably have a headache, or if you are prone to it, a backache. Of course, the party is a success and your acute anxieties were unfounded. Your head- or backache was caused not by the party but by your imaginary fears about it being a disaster.

Similarly, being held up in a traffic jam on your way to work, seeing brown-enveloped bills on your door mat, and having a row with your partner are all events that can bring on backache if you let your imagination take over. For example, you may imagine that you will lose your job because you are late for work, that you will not be able to pay your bills and will end up in a debtor's gaol, and that your partner will walk out on you. All these consequences are highly unlikely and you would be far better off if you did not dwell on them.

Another common example of how easily the body can be misled is shown by viewers' responses to what they watch on television or at the cinema. For example, if you are watching a horror film, your body may respond as if you are really frightened. The hairs on your arms may stand on end, you may feel shivery and your throat may feel dry. You are, of course, not in any danger at all. Your body is responding, not to reality, but to what it *thinks* is happening.

Most of us are constantly creating images and scenarios for ourselves simply by thinking about things. Invariably we then respond to the images and scenarios we have created.

Exactly how your imagination manages to exert this remarkable power over your body is still something of a mystery. But to a large extent the 'how' is academic. The indisputable fact is that, although we may not know exactly how the human mind works, we know that it will respond to scenes it has imagined just as positively and as dramatically as it will respond to reality. Worrying is never good for anyone. But you can, in fact, learn to stop the negative use of your imagination and, instead, put it to good use by deliberately creating peaceful images in your mind.

It may take some time to learn how to do this, but once mastered, it is an easy and very effective procedure which will keep you relaxed and stress free.

For example, try this:

Close your eyes.

Imagine it is a warm sunny day in early summer. The sky is clear blue and cloudless and there is a soft gentle breeze in the air which stops the heat from burning and the day from being oppressive.

It is a perfect day and for a few minutes you can forget all your fears and worries. You are on a private island; alone, content and away from all everyday pressures and stresses. You are alone but not lonely. Around you the world is quiet, but the silence is soothing. Occasionally the breeze rustles the leaves in the nearby trees, and in the distance you can hear insects in the grass and the splash of the waves on the shore.

You walk along a winding track, knowing that no one will ever disturb you here. This is your personal world. No one else can come onto your island without your permission. As you head down the track you gradually become aware that you can hear a stream nearby. It is quite shallow but the water runs fast and is sparkling and crystal clear. Standing on the far side of the stream there is a group of sturdy but old and gnarled trees. Beneath them, in the shade, is a soft and inviting mossy bank. You stand for a few more moments and stare at what seems to you to be the most beautiful and peaceful spot in the world. If you turn to your left you can see the stream meandering down the gently sloping hillside. If you turn to the right you can see where the stream trickles down between rocks and across a stretch of soft golden sand, to the sea.

Using half a dozen large stepping stones you cross the stream, sit down on the mossy bank and rest your back against a tree.

It is like sitting in the most comfortable armchair ever designed. You rest alone, content and silent. You feel comfortable, rested and happy.

When you close your eyes you can hear the clear water of the stream gurgling and bubbling over its rocky bed. In the distance you can hear the sea crashing majestically on the rocks which fringe the island. Above you the breeze is rustling the leaves of the tree you are leaning up against.

You can feel the warmth of the sun filtering down through the leaves and your whole body feels relaxed. You love this peaceful spot.

You can stay here for as long as you wish to. It is your island, your hideaway, your private escape from the real world. Here you can rest, completely untroubled by anxieties.

This sort of simple relaxation technique isn't difficult to learn. But it is an excellent way to combat stress and to defeat anxiety.

RELAX YOUR MIND WITH A DAYDREAM

Close your eyes. Breathe in as slowly as you can. Take big, deep breaths and imagine it is mid morning on a beautiful, warm summer's day.

Imagine that you are standing on a grassy bank, fairly high above the sea. The grass is short and springy and walking on it is like walking on an endless green mattress. You can, if you like, imagine that someone is with you with whom you have such a good relationship that there is no need to talk, someone in whose silent presence you feel comfortable and comforted.

Below and in front of you there are a number of green and fragrant-smelling bushes, alive with the colour of their summer flowers. Just a little way beyond them are rocks and rock pools; beyond the rocks there is a sandy beach, and beyond that there is the sea.

The sea is deep and beautiful blue, broken only by neat lines of white spray where waves are building up and crashing on to the shore. In the distance you can just see two small sailing boats zig-zagging from side to side to make the most of the breeze. There are one or two windsurfers too, though there is so little breeze that they are having to work hard to stay upright. Half a dozen swimmers are bobbing in the clear blue water, clearly enjoying themselves.

You can just hear the sounds of children playing on the beach and splashing about in the shallow water. Several of them are building a sandcastle. They have brightly coloured plastic buckets and spades and are dressed in equally brightly coloured swimsuits. High, high above you half a dozen sea gulls are circling and

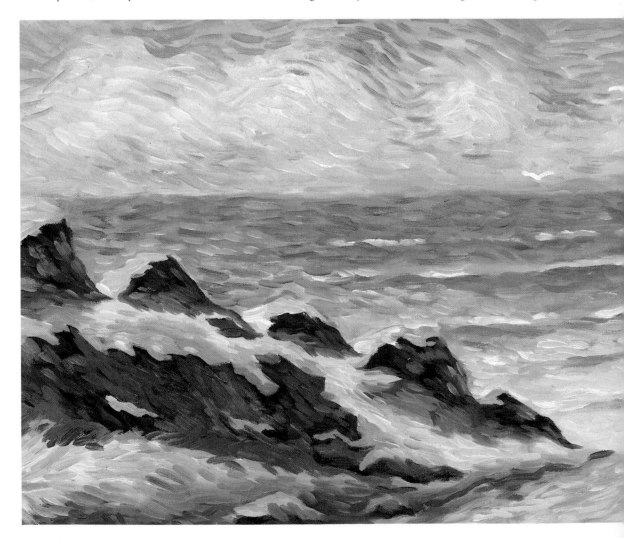

116

calling to one another as they swoop and dive in endless play. The light warm breeze gently caresses your skin and your face and you can just taste the salt of a little sea spray on your lips.

To your left there is a tiny, sandy path. It is almost hidden by a couple of bushes but it looks exciting and inviting so you squeeze between the bushes and follow it as it twists and turns down towards the beach. You are carrying a bag that contains a large, thick bath towel, something to read and a delicious picnic and you use the bag to push aside the bushes so that the branches will not scratch you.

To begin with you expect that the path will lead you down to the large sandy beach that you could see from the top of the hill. But soon you realize that despite its twists and turns the path is heading to the left of where you were standing and cannot possibly be

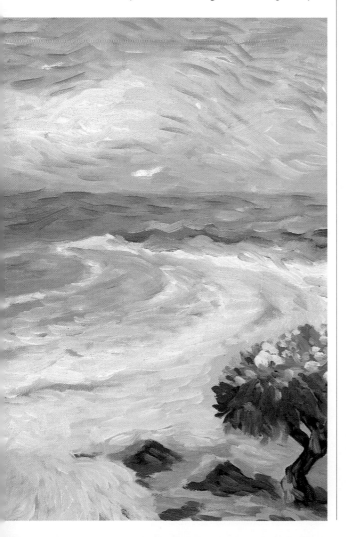

heading for the main beach. You are fascinated and intrigued and your sense of curiosity is aroused.

You walk on and suddenly you turn a sharp corner and there ahead you see where the path is leading. Before you is a beautiful, small private beach. The sand is soft and golden and the beach is surrounded by rocks. It is the most idyllic spot imaginable and it is deserted. Despite the path it is easy to imagine that no one has ever been here before.

You walk down the last few yards of the path until it leads you on to the sand and then you walk slowly across the beach. The sun is warm and apart from the singing of a few birds hidden in the bushes there is nothing but silence around you.

When you lie back you can feel the sun's warm rays on your body and through the towel beneath you the heat rises from the sand. The heat is not uncomfortable or stifling. It is soothing, calming and restful. High, high above you those same few seagulls are circling and calling to one another. You can hear the sound of the waves arriving on the shore too, though there is hardly any breeze here in your small and very private cove. The waves are small and they land on the sand with surprising delicacy.

You close your eyes and all your worries, fears and anxieties seem a million miles away. The heat from the sun above you and the sand below warm your body and you can feel your muscles relaxing. As each moment goes by you become more and more relaxed. You feel comfortable and slightly sleepy. Your muscles are soothed and warm. Your mind is empty of all anxieties. All your worries are set aside for now.

As you lie there on your private beach, on that wonderful summery day, you can feel your whole body relaxing and becoming calm. Your back no longer aches, your muscles and joints are all relaxed and you feel increasingly calm and contented.

And what makes this private place so special is the fact that you can take it with you wherever you go. This is your passport to peace and contentment.

MAKE YOUR OWN DAYDREAMING TAPE

Record the above script so that you can listen to it whenever you need to relax.

Twenty Questions Backache Sufferers Often Ask

Q I LOVE GARDENING BUT HAVE BACKACHE. SHOULD I GIVE IT UP?

A No. Exercise will help strengthen your muscles and keep you fit and healthy. But you will have to be sensible and make some adjustments. When you lift do so with care. Don't bend over to pull out a weed but either use a long-handled tool or bend your knees and keep your back straight. Don't spend hours at a time digging; use a small spade and move little amounts of earth at a time. Change your working position as often as you can, and arrange your garden so that you have as many beds and tubs at waist level as you possibly can. Install a hose or an automatic watering system so that you don't have to carry heavy buckets or watering cans of water around. Kneel or squat instead of bending when you are planting seeds. Plan your garden carefully with lots of ground cover plants to cut down the maintenance work. Wear warm and waterproof clothing in cold weather, and always wear shoes and gloves that don't slip. Rest before you feel tired – don't wait until you ache.

Q MY HUSBAND SUFFERS FROM CHRONIC BACKACHE. I WORRY ABOUT US MAKING LOVE BECAUSE I DON'T WANT TO MAKE HIS BACK WORSE. BECAUSE I'M WORRYING, I CAN'T ENJOY SEX VERY MUCH. WHICH POSITIONS WOULD PUT LEAST STRAIN ON HIS BACK AND BE LEAST LIKELY TO CAUSE PROBLEMS?

A To a certain extent only your husband can know which position is best for him – so you must talk about this together. He needs to be in a position which he

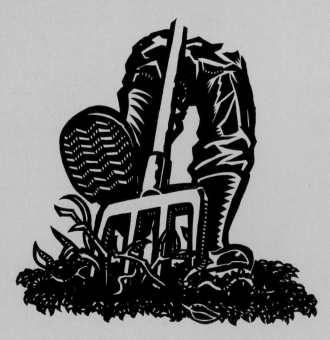

finds comfortable and where there is least strain on his back. If your husband finds the missionary position (where he lies on top of you) uncomfortable then you might find it best if you try the 'woman on top' position. Get your husband to lie down on his back and then kneel astride and above him with your knees either side of his hips. Gently lower yourself onto him from above. This is the least assertive position for a man and requires very little movement. You will be in charge and will be able to control the pace of your love-making. If either or both of you find that position uncomfortable then you could try the 'rear entry

position'. You kneel down and put your hands on the floor, keeping your back horizontal to the floor. Your husband then kneels down and approaches you from behind. He can keep his back fairly straight and there should be very little strain on it in this position. If you find this position tiring you can try building up a pile of cushions or pillows underneath you as support. Alternatively, you can kneel on the floor with your chest resting on a bed or chair.

Q Is it true that the wrong sort of shoes can cause backache? I am quite short and have always worn high-heeled shoes. Could they be responsible for my back trouble?

A Yes. Shoes are a common cause of backache among women, simply because they are more vulnerable to the whims of fashion designers than are men. High-heeled shoes can cause back trouble in four ways. First, they inevitably cause a certain amount of instability when you walk – however good your balance may be – and that instability leads to wobbling, which leads to muscle strains and muscle tension. Backache is then almost inevitable. Second, high heels cause your Achilles tendons to tighten up – and that leads to pain in your calves and, eventually, your back. Third, and probably most important of all, high-heeled shoes offer no protection against jarring when you walk on hard surfaces. Shoes with some bounce in the sole provide a considerable amount of protection against jarring, but high-heeled shoes transmit a shock up your spine every time you move. Finally, high-heeled shoes tend to be rather narrow and tight-fitting, and to produce bunions and other foot problems. People with bad feet tend to have some difficulty in walking – and that puts an additional strain on the whole of the back. Try to keep high-heeled shoes for very special occasions and to wear low-heeled, well-fitting shoes with good 'cushioned' soles for everyday use.

Q What is scoliosis?

A Scoliosis is a sideways or lateral bend or curve in the spine that may be inherited and may be due to some congenital problem. It is most common in children. It can be caused by muscle spasm which has been caused

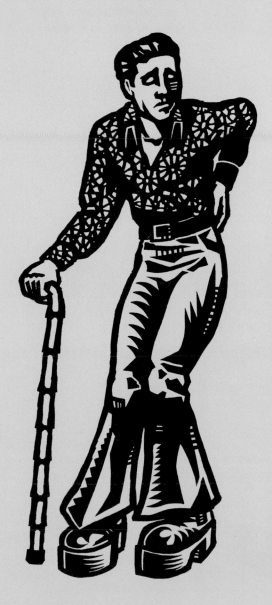

by overstretching of ligaments and muscles on one side of the back. Always carrying heavy shopping in the same hand or always carrying a shoulder bag on the same side can cause scoliosis in adults. Sometimes scoliosis develops because an individual's legs are of different lengths, but the difference has to be quite large to cause a noticeable problem; one in ten men and women have a difference in leg length of at least a centimetre and relatively few ever notice anything. Mild scoliosis doesn't usually produce much, if any, pain to begin with, but as the years go by the unequal strains and stresses can put a strain on the joints in the spine and result in backache. Very occasionally, a deformity in the spine is so great that surgery is needed to straighten things out. When children are affected by scoliosis a brace may need to be worn to keep the spine as straight as possible.

Q MY DOCTOR IS TRYING SOME NEW PAINKILLERS OUT ON ME, BUT I FIND IT DIFFICULT TO BE PRECISE ABOUT WHETHER OR NOT THEY ARE HELPING. I HAVE DIFFICULTY IN SAYING FOR CERTAIN WHETHER MY PAIN IS WORSE TODAY THAN IT WAS, SAY, LAST WEEK OR LAST MONTH. IS THERE ANY DEVICE AVAILABLE THAT WILL MEASURE PAIN ACCURATELY?

A Try using an ordinary school ruler. The left-hand edge of the ruler marks complete freedom from pain. The right-hand edge of the ruler marks the worst pain that you can possibly imagine. Simply look carefully at the ruler and decide just where on that scale your pain should be measured. And then make a note of the reading you have taken. On subsequent occasions you simply look at your ruler again and make a fresh assessment. You can then measure whether your pain seems to be getting worse, getting better or staying the same. You'll find another technique for measuring pain on page 84.

Q I READ RECENTLY THAT THE AUTHOR ERNEST HEMINGWAY WROTE MANY OF HIS BOOKS WHILE STANDING UP BECAUSE HE SUFFERED FROM BACKACHE. IS STANDING UP BETTER FOR A BAD BACK THAN SITTING DOWN? I WOULD HAVE THOUGHT THAT SITTING TOOK SOME OF THE STRAIN OFF THE BACK.

A If the pressure within the intervertebral discs at the bottom of your spine is 100 per cent when you are standing up straight, it will be 150 per cent when you are sitting up straight in an ordinary dining-type chair, and a massive 250 per cent when you are slouching or slumped forward in a chair. It will be 25 per cent when you are lying flat on your back in bed. In short, standing is much better for your back than sitting, and Ernest Hemingway knew what he was doing.

Q I DO A LOT OF DRIVING AND NEARLY ALWAYS GET OUT OF THE CAR ACHING AND FEELING STIFF. IS THERE ANYTHING I CAN DO TO HELP MY BACK?

A Car seats are, in general, very badly designed, and are responsible for millions of cases of backache. Try to make sure that your car has a seat which can be adjusted in as many ways as possible. The seat should be firm (though not too firm – hard tractor seats cause lots of problems by transmitting vibrations directly up into the spine), and the backrest should give plenty of support. Then adjust the seat so that you feel comfortable and can reach the controls easily and without stretching. If your seat doesn't give your lower back the support it needs buy a cushion to slip or tie behind your back. Try to make sure that you are relaxed while you are driving – don't let yourself get stressed by traffic queues or badly behaved motorists. Learn how to relax your body and your mind (see pages 112-115). Many motorists find having a car radio or cassette player an essential tool for relaxed driving. Stop frequently when driving on long journeys. Get out of the car and walk around for a few minutes.

Q ARE ANY SPORTS PARTICULARLY BAD FOR THE BACK?

A *All* sports are potentially bad for the back. Contact sports such as rugby and judo can cause serious damage to the spine if you fall awkwardly – particularly on hard ground. Running and horse riding can cause problems because of vibrations being transmitted up through the spine. Even golf can cause lots of back trouble – particularly if you swing badly, carry too many clubs or

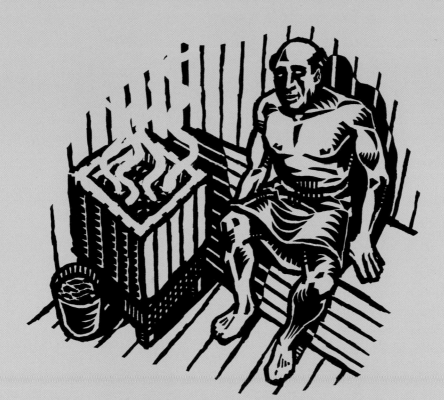

hit the ground with your club. Whatever sport you play, think carefully about potential causes of back trouble and do what you can to avoid problems – rather than waiting for problems to arise.

Q I SUFFER FROM BACK TROUBLE AND REALLY NEED A FIRMER BED, BUT I CAN'T AFFORD ONE. HAVE YOU ANY ADVICE?

A You don't have to buy a special orthopaedic mattress. One possibility is to put a board underneath the length of your mattress to make it firmer. Alternatively, put your mattress, a sleeping bag or a quilt on the floor and sleep on the floor itself – using pillows and cushions to make yourself comfortable and to help keep your back straight.

Q I HAVE HEARD THAT A SAUNA IS GOOD FOR A BAD BACK. IS THIS TRUE?

A It can certainly help a minor back problem. The heat of a sauna encourages the superficial circulation and this helps to get rid of mild aches and pains. A warm bath or shower helps in a similar way.

Q IS BACKACHE AN INEVITABLE RESULT OF AGEING?

A No, there are lots of sprightly 80-year-olds around. Backache gets more common as we get older, but it is not an inevitable consequence of growing older. Exercise regularly (and carefully), keep your weight under control and make sure that your posture is good – particularly while sitting down – and you will reduce the risk of developing back trouble.

Q DO YOU KNOW OF ANY HERBAL REMEDIES WHICH CAN BE USED FOR THE TREATMENT OF BACKACHE?

A I know of many herbal remedies which are recommended for the treatment of backache – but personally I do not recommend any of them. In general herbal products have all the disadvantages of modern drugs (plus the additional risk of impurity and accidental toxicity), and few of the advantages. Many modern drugs are derived from plants. The aspirin tablet, for example, comes from the willow tree, while morphine comes from the opium poppy.

Q WHAT IS A FUTON?

A This is a thin but firm mattress popular in Japan for several thousand years. At bedtime a futon is rolled out on the floor or on a base frame to provide a comfortable but fairly solid bed that many backache sufferers find very suitable.

Q CAN TIREDNESS CAUSE BACKACHE? I FIND THAT MY BACK TROUBLE IS WORSE WHEN I HAVE BEEN WORKING HARD.

A Exhaustion means strained, stressed and tired muscles. Backache is often one of the first symptoms which show that you need to rest.

Q IS A DESK THAT IS FLAT BETTER OR WORSE THAN A DESK THAT SLOPES?

A A writing slope – such as was popular a century or so ago in schools and offices – is much better for your back than a flat desk. A horizontal surface creates back problems since it encourages too much bending of the back. A Victorian writing slope encourages the user to sit properly – particularly if used with a traditional stool. We often think that we have improved our world since the 19th century but in many ways progress and new technology have just made it worse. It is hardly surprising that backache is endemic.

Q I SUFFER FROM BACK TROUBLE AND GET PINS AND NEEDLES IN MY LEG. WHAT CAUSES IT?

A The tingling feeling known as pins and needles is caused when a nerve is compressed. Your doctor should be able to tell which nerve is being compressed – and where – by the position of your pins and needles.

Q MY UNCLE IS IN THE ARMY AND CLAIMS THAT AN ERECT 'MILITARY' POSTURE IS BEST FOR AVOIDING BACK TROUBLE. IS HE RIGHT?

A I'm afraid he isn't – if by a 'military' posture he means standing with his shoulders pushed back and his bottom pushed right out in a rather exaggerated way. A 'military' posture can lead to back problems almost as easily as a sloppy, distinctly 'unmilitary' posture.

Q WHY DOES PREGNANCY SO OFTEN CAUSE BACKACHE AMONG WOMEN? AND WHAT CAN BE

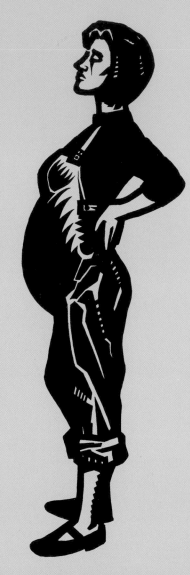

DONE TO REDUCE THE RISK OF BACKACHE DEVELOPING? I HAVE JUST BECOME PREGNANT AND AM KEEN TO REDUCE THE RISK OF A PROBLEM DEVELOPING.

A There are several factors that make backache more likely during pregnancy. First, of course, there is the developing bulge at the front. This puts a tremendous strain on the joints of the back and changes the centre of gravity. Ten pounds of excess weight carried on your abdomen is equivalent to a pressure of 100 lb of additional weight inside your spine. As your abdomen gets bigger so your spine gets pushed more and more out of shape. Second, just to make things worse, your body will produce a hormone during pregnancy which is designed to soften and stretch the ligaments at the bottom of your spine so that your baby can be delivered more easily. The combination of extra weight and weaker ligaments makes backache a virtual inevitability. However, there are several things you can do to limit the risks of back trouble developing. Exercise regularly, make sure that your weight does not rise more than it needs to, avoid bending, learn to lift properly, avoid carrying heavy loads (use a trolley or a basket on wheels for shopping), rest regularly, attend antenatal classes to learn suitable exercises and wear flat or low-heeled shoes since high, narrow heels will simply make things worse.

Q CAN COLD DRAUGHTS CAUSE BACK TROUBLE?

A Yes. Cold draughts or winds cause trouble by making muscles cold and encouraging them to go into spasm. Avoid sitting or standing in draughts and wear warm clothes if you have to go out into the cold.

Q WHAT IS HYDROTHERAPY? AND HOW CAN IT HELP BACKACHE?

A Hydrotherapy simply means 'treatment in or with water' and it has always been popular. Both the Greeks and the Romans believed in the therapeutic powers of bathing, as did many primitive societies in the curative powers of Holy Wells and springs. In the 18th century 'taking the waters' was popular at spa towns all over Europe. Today there has been a revival in the popularity of spas. In Britain spa towns such as Bath, Harrogate and Leamington are popular; in Germany back sufferers flock to resorts such as Baden Baden, and in France thousands of treatments a day are given in Vichy alone. Hydrotherapy can mean drinking water, splashing it onto your body, bathing in it, sitting in it, swimming in it and exercising in it. The water can be used cold, warm or hot. It can be delivered by hose, bucket or drinking glass. The dangers are limited. Public baths and whirlpools can produce or exacerbate urinary problems such as cystitis, and water that is too hot can scald. But swimming and exercising in warm water can help relieve and prevent joint, bone or muscle troubles – including backache, of course.

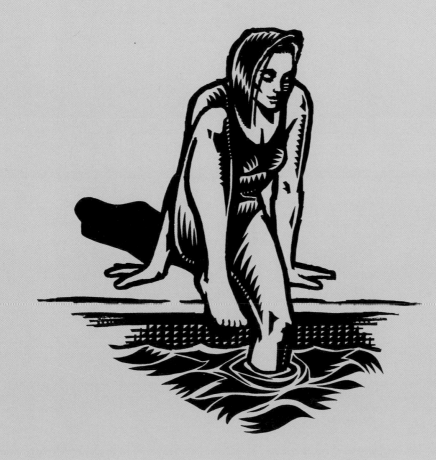

Appendix

AIDS FOR BACKACHE SUFFERERS

Because of stiffness in their spines backache sufferers often have difficulty in bending and reaching. To help overcome these problems there are many commercially available products which reduce the need for bending, reaching and lifting, and which help to protect the back and prevent the development of problems.

This appendix does not attempt to offer a comprehensive list of aids for backache sufferers but is designed to show the range available. You should be able to obtain a full list from your family doctor or hospital consultant, but if you have any difficulty I suggest that you contact one of the many charitable or commercial organizations offering aids for the disabled. Large towns often have shops which specialize in offering equipment designed to make life easier for backache sufferers.

AIDS FOR SITTING

POSTURE STOOL

The seat slopes forwards and you sit with your weight resting on your knees and your feet tucked in underneath you. The posture stool is designed to encourage you to sit in a healthier position so that you can get up at the end of a day's work without having a stiff and aching back.

BACKRESTS, 'WEDGES' AND LUMBAR SUPPORTS

Most chairs do not provide enough support for the lumbar part of the spine. You can buy many different supports – including inflatable cushions which are suitable for travellers – which will help turn your uncomfortable chair into one which is much friendlier to your back.

ADJUSTABLE CHAIRS

Properly adjustable chairs which allow you to sit in a comfortable position are available, but they do tend to be expensive. The seat height should be adjustable, as should the angle of the seat and the backrest. You'll find it easier to get into and out of chairs which have arm rests that you can rest your weight on when sitting down or push against when standing up. If your feet aren't resting on the floor when you are sitting down then you need a footrest (dangling feet add to the stress on your spine).

EJECTOR CHAIRS

It is possible to buy chairs which, at the touch of a lever, help to push you up into the standing position.

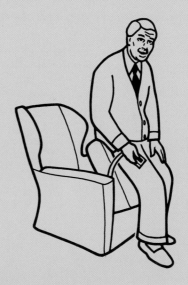

AIDS FOR WORK

WRITING SLOPES

If you work on a computer, word processor or typewriter you may need to have a flat desk. But writing slopes enable you to work at an angle which is better suited to your body.

TIP FOR SURVIVING AT WORK

Get up and walk about every half an hour or so. This will give you a chance to stretch your back and will help prevent muscle, joint and ligament strain.

AIDS FOR PICKING THINGS UP

Simple 'pick up sticks' (such as are often used by park attendants employed to pick up bits and pieces of waste paper) help make life much easier if you find it difficult to bend or to reach for small objects. With a little experience you will find that a pick up stick extends your reach by three feet and enables you to pick up all sorts of things (clothes, books, magazines, newspapers, rubbish etc.) off the floor without bending down.

AIDS IN THE GARDEN

Use a smaller fork or spade to limit the load on your back when digging. Use long-handled tools and shears to help you garden without bending, reaching, stooping or stretching for long periods. Don't overload wheelbarrows. Use raised beds whenever possible so that you can do as much gardening as possible without bending down. If you have to get down to ground level kneel on a mat.

WALKING AIDS

If you have difficulty in walking and your doctor recommends one don't be too proud to use a walking stick or frame to give you extra support, to take some of the strain and to allow you to rest when you need to. If you use a stick make sure it has a non-stick end, and change hands regularly so that you don't get into the habit of putting too much strain on one side of your body. Walking frames can be equipped with baskets so that you don't have to carry bags.

AIDS FOR SHOPPING

If you have to carry heavy loads around use a shopping trolley or basket on wheels to relieve the strain on your back. Recent research from France showed that the average six-year-old French child regularly carries nine per cent of his or her own body-weight in a rucksack or satchel while travelling to and from school. By the age of 12 the load has risen to 25 per cent and by the time they reach 16 years of age pupils are carrying 50 per cent of their body-weight around with them in books, sports gear etc. It is hardly surprising that in the last decade the number of French citizens suffering from severe back problems has risen from 30 per cent to 45 per cent.

AIDS FOR GETTING UP AND DOWN STAIRS

If you find walking up and down stairs painful you may find it easier if you edge yourself up or down stairs on your bottom.

If your problem persists, investigate the possibility of installing a powered stair lift. You sit down on a small chair, press a button and ascend or descend the stairs effortlessly.

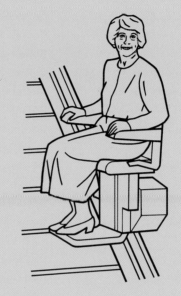

AIDS FOR GETTING DRESSED

If you have difficulty in bending or raising your arms, you will find that some clothes are far more difficult to get into and out of than others. Avoid tight jeans or trousers. Wear slip on shoes rather than lace-ups. Make sure that zips and buttons are easily accessible, and replace difficult to reach and difficult to use fasteners with easy-to-reach and easy-to-use fasteners. Velcro fastenings are easy to close and undo.

TIPS FOR DRESSING

1. Lean against a wall when you need to raise a foot or leg (e.g. to put on a sock or tie a shoelace)
2. Roll up clothes (e.g. jumpers) so that you can put your arms through the arm holes as easily as possible
3. If you have difficulty in balancing or pulling on trousers or tights try dressing while lying on top of your bed. To get your trousers over your feet pull your knees up to your chest. Then straighten your legs to pull your trousers up to your bottom.

BACKACHE INDEX

Abdomen 11

Acetylsalicylic acid 76

Acupuncture 25, 100, 103

Aerobics 63-64

Age/pulse range 61

Ageing 18-19

Alexander, F. Matthias 104

Alexander Technique 104-105

Alternative practitioners 102
  How to choose 102

Alternative therapy 100-109

Ankylosing spondylitis 13, 15

Annulus fibrosus 10

Anxiety 46

Arachnoiditis 15, 27

Arthritis 13, 14, 33, 46, 103

Aspirin 76, 78, 79

Asthma 33

Atlas bone
  see Vertebrae

Axis bone
  see Vertebrae

Backache aids and helps 124-125

Back injury, causes of 20-21, 28, 46

Back pain 70
  Tips on how to avoid 28, 46, 118-125
  Tips on beds 32

Benzodiazepine
  see Tranquillizers

Blood pressure, high 33

Blood vessels 10

Brain 8

Caffeine 90

Callisthenics 62

Cancer of the spine 18

Cerebro-spinal fluid 11

Cervical spine 12

Cervical vertebrae
  see Vertebrae

Chiropractic 25, 105

Chymopapain
  see Injections

Circulation problems 46

Coccygeal region 9

Coccyx 8

Codeine 78, 79

Collars 75

Compressed nerves 72, 122

Corsets 75

Corticosteroid 75, 76
  see Steroids

CT-scan 25, 27

Daydream tape 116-117

Decompression surgery 27, 72

Degenerative changes (growing old) 18-20
  Of disc 20
  Of joint 20
  Of ligament 20

Depression 33, 46, 98

Descartes 96

Diabetes mellitus 33

Digestive upsets 46

Discectomy 72

Discography 25, 26

Discs
  Intervertebral 8, 10
  Prolapsed or slipped 8, 12, 13, 22, 72

Dressing tips 125

Driving and back pain 120

Drugs, prescribed dosage 80-81

Dysmenorrhoea 16

Eczema 33

Electromyography 27

Endometriosis 18

Endorphins 79

Enkephalins 79

Epidural
  see Injections

Exercise 11, 30, 44-46
  Aerobic 61-64
  Dangerous 59
  Flexibility 65
  Mobilizing 25
  Muscle development 66-69
  Stretching 54-57
  Strengthening 47, 53

Exercises for backs 44, 47-58

Fibroids 16

Fibrous capsule 22

Fractured bones 72

Galen 78

Gall stones 18, 33

Gardening and back trouble 118

Gate control theory 84, 97

Gynaecological problems 13, 16

Hahnemann, Samuel 108

Headaches 46

Healing 105

Heat pain relief 86

Heart disease 18, 33, 46

Herbalists 100

Hernia 33

Heroin 79

Hip bones 9

Hippocrates 78, 108

Homeopathy 100, 108

Hydrotherapy 103, 123

Ibuprofen 76

Ice pain relief 87

Imagination 92

Indigestion 18

Indomethacin 76

Inferior articular process
  see Processes
Injections 75
  Chymopapain 76
  Epidural 76
  Sclerosant (Prolotherapy) 75
  Steroid 75
Interferential therapy 75
Intestines 10
Irritable bowel syndrome 16, 17, 46
Isometrics 62

Kennedy, President John F. 92
Kidney infection 13
Kidney stone 13, 18
Kinins 96
Krieger, Dolores 107

Lifting techniques 28, 30
Ligaments 6, 10, 12, 20
Lumbar vertebrae
  see Vertebrae
Lumbar supports 124

Malaria 108
Manipulation 73
Massage 88
Mefanamic acid 76
Melzack, Ronald and Wall, Patrick 84, 97
Meningitis 12, 15
Mobilization 25, 73
Morphine 76, 78, 79
  see Opiates
Muscle development
  see Exercise
Muscles 6
  Involuntary 10
  Voluntary 10-11
Myelography 25, 27

Neck 12
Nerves 8, 11

Neural arch 9, 11
Nucleus polposus 8, 10, 22

Obesity 30, 46
  see Weight loss
Opiates 78-79
Osteitis deformans 15
Osteoarthritis 12, 13, 14
Osteomalacia 14
Osteopathy 25, 100, 109
Osteoporosis 13, 14
Oxygen 11, 62

Pain 70, 96
Painful periods 16
Painkillers 80
  How to take 80, 81
Pain measurement 84, 120
Pain relief 80, 82
  Heat 86
  Ice 87
  Imagination and control techniques 92-93
  Massage 88
  Music 87
  TENS 85
  Vibration 86
Paget's disease 15
Pancreatitis 18
Paracelsus 108
Paracetamol 76
Paralysis 6, 8
Pelvis 6
Phenybutazone 76
Physiotherapy 73
Piles 33
Pinched nerve 26, 122
Pleurisy 12
Pneumonia 12, 18
Posture 12, 21, 122
Pregnancy 122
Processes 9
  Inferior articular 9
  Spinous 9, 11
  Superior articular 9

Transverse 9, 11
Prolapsed disc
  see Disc
Prolapsed womb 18
Prolotherapy
  see Injections
Prostaglandins 76, 96

Quinine 108

Relaxation 91, 110
  Daydream 116-117
  Techniques 112-114
Relaxation tape 114
Retroverted uterus 16
Rheumatoid arthritis 14
Ribs 9

Sacral bones 9
Sacral region 9
Sacral vertebrae
  see Vertebrae
Sacrum 8, 24
Sacroiliac joint strain 13
Sciatica 13, 24
Scoliosis 119
Sex and back trouble 118
Shaw, George Bernard 81
Shingles 18
Shoes 119
Short-wave diathermy 75
Skull 8, 9
Sleep 32
Sleeplessness 46
Slipped disc
  see Discs
Spinal canal 11
Spinal cord 6, 8, 11, 22, 97
Spine 6, 8, 9
Spinous process
  see Processes
Steroids 75
  see Injections
  Side effects 75
Still, Andrew Taylor 109

Stomach ulcer 13, 18

Strained muscles 13

Stress 12, 15

Strokes 33

Superior articular process
  see Processes

Surgery 27, 72-73
  Decompression 27, 72
  Discectomy 72
  Spinal fusion 72

Surrey University 28

Swimming, benefits of 60

Tendons 6

TENS (Transcutaneous nerve
  stimulation) 75, 84-86

Thin bones 13

Thoracic Vertebrae
  see Vertebrae

Traction 73

Tranquillizers 78, 79

Transverse processes
  see Processes

Tumours 72

Ultrasound 75

Varicose veins 33

Vertebrae 6, 8, 72
  Atlas bone 10
  Axis bone 10
  Cervical 8, 9, 10
  Lumbar 8, 9, 24
  Sacral 8
  Thoracic 8, 9

Vertebral column 11

Vibrator 86

Virus infection 15

Weight/height chart 43

Weight loss 32-39
  Slimming tape 39
  Slimming tips 40-42

Whiplash syndrome 12

World Health Organization
  103

X-rays 25, 26

PHOTOGRAPHIC ACKNOWLEDGEMENTS

The photographs in this book are from the following sources:

Andes Press Agency, London/Carlos Reyes 71; Camera Press, London/Jungkwan Chi 101; J. Allan Cash Photolibrary, London 74; Sally and Richard Greenhill, London 19; Institute of Orthopaedics, University College London 27; Sylvia Pitcher, London 91; Reed International Books/Alex Williams 29; Rex Features Limited, London: Hutchings 104, Gueorgui Pinkhassov/Sipa Press 81; Science Photo Library, London/Simon Fraser/Hexham General 85; Edwin Smith, Saffron Walden; Frank Spooner Pictures, London/Eric Bouvet/Gamma 45; Tony Stone Photolibrary, London: Bruce Ayres 34, Chris Lane 37; Telegraph Colour Library, London/Stock Directory 33; ZEFA, London: R. Bond 111, Sharp Shooters/M. Vaughn 94, H. Sochurek 23

SPECIAL PHOTOGRAPHY

Richard Truscott 2, 4, 7, 12, 31, 48 (all four), 49 (all four), 50 (all three), 51 (all three), 52 (all four), 53 (all four), 54 (all four), 55 (all four), 56 (all four), 57 (all four), 58 (all four), 66 (all four) 67 (all four), 68 (all four), 69 left and right

ILLUSTRATION

Malcolm Chandler 116

LINE ARTWORK

Jared Gibey 8, 9, 10, 24, 124, 125
Simon David 118, 119, 121, 122, 123

DESIGN/ART DIRECTION Sarah Pollock
EDITOR Sian Facer
PRODUCTION Alison Myer
PICTURE RESEARCH Judy Todd